Pertussis & Whooping Cough

Pertussis & Whooping Cough Care & Treatment

Including: Pertussis & Whooping Cough Vaccine, Bordetella Pertussis, Acellular Pertussis, Natural Remedies, Symptoms, Treatment, Diagnosis

Agatha Harding, APRN.

Copyright © 2024

Copyright and Trademarks

All rights reserved. No part of this book may be reproduced or transferred in any form or by any means without written permission of the publisher and author. This publication is Copyright Protected. All products, publications, software and services mentioned in this publication are protected by trademarks.

Disclaimer and Legal Notice

This product is not legal, accounting, medical or health advice and should not be interpreted in that manner. You need to do your own due-diligence to determine if the content of this book is right for you. While we have tried our very best to verify the information in this publication, neither the authors, publisher nor the affiliates assume any responsibility for errors, omissions or contrary interpretation of the subject matter herein.

We have no control over the nature, content and availability of the web sites, products or sources listed in this book. The inclusion of any web site links does not necessarily imply a recommendation or endorsement of the views expressed within them. Ocean Blue Publishing and the authors take no responsibility nor will they be liable for the websites or content being unavailable or removed.

The advice and strategies contained herein may not be suitable for every individual. The authors and publisher shall not be liable for any loss incurred as a consequence of the use and/or the application, directly or indirectly, of any information presented in this work. This publication is designed to provide information in regard to the subject matter covered.

Neither the authors nor the publisher assume any responsibility for any errors or omissions, nor do they represent or warrant that the information, ideas, plans, actions, suggestions and methods of operation contained herein is in all cases true, accurate, appropriate, or legal. It is the reader's responsibility to consult with an appropriate medical professional before putting any of the enclosed information, ideas, or practices written in this book in to practice.

Acknowledgements

Thank you to the many around the world that helped in contributing with insights and experiences of living and coping with this condition. We very much appreciate your input. It is your support that has helped in making this a resourceful book that will no doubt help others around the world.

I'd also like to thank my family for their continued love and support through this journey.

Finally I would like to wish a strong recovery and good health to all those that suffer from any type of illness or condition. Our thoughts are with you.

Table of Contents

INTRODUCTION — 4

CHAPTER ONE: WHAT IS WHOOPING COUGH? — 6

CHAPTER TWO: CAUSES — 19

CHAPTER THREE: TRADITIONAL TREATMENTS — 33

CHAPTER FOUR: PROS AND CONS OF VACCINATIONS — 42

CHAPTER FIVE: TREATING WHOOPING COUGH — 93

Introduction

Pertussis, more commonly known as whooping cough, is a contagious infection that affects mostly children. It is identified by professionals and laypeople alike by the severe fits of coughing that typically end in a whooping sound. Many parents remark that this sound can be described as high pitched, prolonged, and deeply in-drawn breath.

Whooping cough was once a rather prevalent and rampant disease not only in the United States but around the world. Today, although less prevalent than in the past, the disease still affects many people, especially in third world countries where vaccinations are not as readily available.

However, despite the fact that many childhood diseases and conditions, including Pertussis, in developed countries have been relatively uncommon during the past few decades, they are making a resurgence due to the fact that increasing numbers of parents are opting not to vaccinate their children for common childhood diseases – for a variety of reasons.

We will be covering the pros and cons about vaccinations. Disagreements regarding school requirements to vaccinate prior to admission are common and prevalent throughout the United States and developed countries around the world today.

History has taught us lessons, and we'll provide a brief glimpse of what whooping cough was like before vaccinations were offered. Finally, we'll provide information regarding holistic or alternative approaches to treating whooping cough as well as the use of antibiotics - and the safety and efficacy of conventional or traditional treatments and alternative forms of treatment for whooping cough.

Our intention is to provide unbiased information for parents regarding this disease, and the pros and cons of vaccinations and vaccine schedules that are backed by verifiable research. We will also mention some of the misinformation and myths regarding some of these topics so that you can make informed and rational decisions whether to vaccinate or not.

We're going to tell you exactly what is in these vaccines and how these components work throughout the development, manufacturing, and delivery process.

Only when you know what is in these vaccines and their effects can you make that informed and knowledgeable decision regarding immunization without having to decide only on innuendo, myth, and misinformation. Get the facts first.

We'll talk about how pertussis is transmitted, and the occurrence of cases based on geographical locations, as well as presenting a brief history of the illness. Parents should know the signs and symptoms of the illness and when to see a doctor. Understanding the different stages of the illness that can occur is also important for parents seeking the best treatment for whooping cough.

Most importantly, we encourage every parent to research not only the topic of pertussis or whooping cough, but also all common childhood diseases.

Information will empower you. Use accurate and scientifically proven research when making such decisions. If, after reading this book, you have additional questions or concerns, please feel free to let us know. We'll help you find the answers you are looking for.

Chapter One: What is Whooping Cough?

A Brief History

The condition "whooping cough" was originally identified in France in the 1500s. Back then, it was called "the dog bark" disease. At that time, while it affected all age groups, it was often fatal for younger children and older people. In the past, the disease killed thousands on a yearly basis, and still does in countries where the vaccine is not readily available.

Whooping cough or pertussis, as described in the introduction, is very contagious. The disease is caused by the Bordetella pertussis bacterium. It's classified as an aerobic organism, meaning that it requires oxygen to survive.

Up until the twentieth century, the disease was particularly dangerous and virulent but with the advent of vaccines, it decreased in scope to the point of eradication – but now is making a comeback. More on that will be covered later.

Humans are the only carriers of the Bordetella pertussis bacteria, which needs warm conditions to survive (such as that provided by the human body).

Localized epidemics may occur every three to five years. While the condition can develop at any age, many cases occur in children under five years of age. In older people, the disease is often milder or asymptomatic, but they are usually the source of infection for infants and children.

Today, pertussis and cases of "walking pneumonia" are often confused and misdiagnosed. However, before getting into details about the cause of the disease, its progression, and pros and cons of vaccination, as well as treatments, it should be noted that pertussis can be very serious and even fatal among children under two years of age.

Pertussis has been around for centuries, with earliest reports of the disease dating back to the 12th century. It was first named and described in literature in 1578, but it wasn't until 1906 that the actual bacterial microbe was isolated in a culture by Octave Gengou and Jules Bordet. Pertussis, as a term to define the disease, has been recognized since the 18th century.

In 1913, a headline for the New York Times newspaper proclaimed "Whooping Cough a Germ Disease". In 1914, the New York Times presented an article titled "Physicians in War on Whooping Cough" that described setting up isolation wards as a recommendation for the treatment of such cases. In that article it was mentioned that in 1913, in New York City, an estimated 500 children fell victim to the disease.

In the early days of treatment options, a number of trial and error methods began, including the use of x-rays to treat the disease (although now it's known that it didn't have any real effects).

Even though Gengou and Bordet identified the bacteria in 1906, it wasn't until the early 1940s that relatively effective treatments and vaccines were offered to the public. The following year, in 1941, the Michigan Department of Health described "favorable" results using the pertussis vaccination available at the time, sometimes by itself and sometimes in combination with the diphtheria vaccination.

In December 1941, the New York Times also released statistics that in that year approximately 6,850 cases in New York City alone had been diagnosed, with 38 deaths as a direct result of the pertussis bacteria.

After the Second World War, cases of pertussis gradually declined, as more effective vaccines were made available to the general public.

It wasn't until the 1990s that the rise in cases of pertussis in the United States began to attract more attention. This culminated in an alarming 25,000 cases in 2005, with a sharp drop-off following the availability of new vaccines that same year.

In 2008, approximately 13,000 pertussis cases or infections throughout the United States were identified, with 19 children (all under the age of one) dying from the disease.

Around the world today, approximately 50 million people are exposed to and experience the symptoms of whooping cough. Every year, and especially in third world countries, hundreds of thousands of people continue to die from it. In fact, in modern times, nearly 9 out of 10 cases of whooping cough occur in third world countries.

Many people believe that whooping cough is only a childhood disease, but it affects teenagers and adults as well. The elderly, especially those 65 years of age or older, are especially vulnerable

when they also have complications from another illness or disease processes.

In the days before vaccines became available, the condition caused the death of 5,000 to 10,000 individuals every year in the United States alone. Because of the pertussis vaccine, the annual death rate today is less than 30 per year, which has been the figure from around 2004.

Since the 1950s, cases of pertussis have steadily increased, spiking in 2005 with the aforementioned 25,000 children being diagnosed. Among this number were infants younger than six months of age who contracted the condition before they were protected by immunization, as well as children between the ages of 11 and 18, whose immunity had waned.

With the uptick of pertussis cases diagnosed in the United States and other developed countries around the world, there is an increase in the number of cases in children around 11 years of age. The commonly held opinion is that this resurgence is mainly because after about the age of 10, vaccines are not necessary anymore.

This coincides with the rough estimate of the duration of protection the pertussis vaccine offers. The increase in socialization and interaction in the early and mid-teen years has also contributed to the number of cases going up overall and within this age group.

One of the common assumptions made by many parents and individuals regarding childhood vaccines is that once you are vaccinated, you are good for life, but this is just not the case.

While vaccines do benefit children greatly by enabling the body to build up antibodies against specific diseases following injection, some vaccines may not provide permanent protection – some vaccines have been quite successful in this regard, such as polio and measles.

Many vaccines need to be updated on a regular basis especially for children. If not, whooping cough can still be contracted later on in life after the initial protection offered by the vaccine has worn off.

In recent years, increasing numbers of cases of pertussis in teenagers and adults have been reported to the Centers for Disease Control and Prevention (CDC). The American Academy of Pediatrics recommends that children between the ages of 11 and 18 get booster shots to help bolster their immunity.

In 2012, the CDC reported that cases of whooping cough/pertussis were at their highest levels in 50 years. The CDC is not the only organization concerned. The National Center for Immunization and Respiratory Diseases reported that a child who remains unvaccinated is at an eight times higher risk of contracting pertussis than a child who has been vaccinated.

Vaccinated children generally experience a milder course of the illness and are less infectious than those who have not if they contract the disease following vaccination.

In 2012, ABC news reported that a pertussis outbreak may be worse in 50 years. Live Science Magazine also reported on the 2012 outbreak, stating that the high number of cases might be due belief that today's vaccination against whooping cough is less effective than those of the past, according to the Professor of Pediatric Infectious Diseases at the David Geffen School of Medicine and the University of California Los Angeles.

In the 1940s, there were approximately 157 cases of pertussis per 100,000 individuals, and during this decade, the whole cell pertussis vaccine was first introduced to the public.

Take a look at some other stats regarding the reduction and near-eradication of the disease over the past few decades:

a) Less than 1 case per 100,000 individuals by 1973

b) Less than 3 cases per 100,000 individuals throughout the 1980s and 1990s

c) 9 cases per 100,000 since 2000 and rising

Outbreaks in the United States in 2005, 2010, and 2012 brought increased awareness regarding the efficacy of vaccines as well as adaptations of vaccines currently under development.

Apparently, studies have determined that the DTaP vaccines today are less effective than the DTP vaccine of the past.

In fact, that earlier version of the vaccine, then called the "whole cell pertussis vaccine", provided extremely long-lasting immunity, which was also believed to last a lifetime. Small reactions of that vaccine included redness and swelling at the injection site.

In the 1990s, a vaccine known as the acellular pertussis vaccine was offered to the public, and was combined with diphtheria and tetanus vaccine, today nicknamed the DTaP vaccine.

Note: To avoid confusion, we need to take a moment to differentiate between the DTaP and the Tdap vaccines. The DTaP (Diphtheria, Tetanus, and Pertussis) is generally given to children under the age of 7. The Tdap (Tetanus, Diphtheria, and Pertussis) vaccine is designed as a booster to be given at or after the age of 11. It can be confusing!

We should also define the difference between the older whole cell pertussis vaccines (also known as the DTwP) and the newer acellular vaccine. The whole cell pertussis vaccine was used for more than six decades, up until the 1980s. The newer acellular vaccines have been used since the early 1990s. The acellular version (chemically detoxified – aka recombinant) was determined to be safer, but does not appear to have the same efficacy as the older version.

In June 2014, California declared a whooping cough epidemic after 800 cases of whooping cough were diagnosed within a three week period, and altogether so far, there were 3,458 cases. According to the American Association of Family Practitioners (AAFP), whooping cough outbreaks have become an increasingly common concern among pediatricians.

The year before, in 2013, approximately 2,530 cases were reported to the California Department of Public Health. In the year 2014 up to the month of June, nearly 10,000 cases of pertussis were reported to the Center for Disease Control by all states in the United States - a 24% increase from the previous year!

In the case of the California epidemic, it was determined that over 80% of the cases occurred in children between the ages of 7 and 16, as well as infants. Nearly 65% of infants under four months of age required hospitalization, with two infant deaths reported.

As a result, the California Department of Public Health urged pregnant women to get their vaccinations. They also urged parents to vaccinate their infants as soon as possible. Pertussis vaccinations do not provide lifetime immunity.

Nevertheless the California Department of Public Health Director at the time, Ron Chapman, suggested that the Tdap (tetanus, diphtheria, and acellular pertussis) booster vaccination was the best way that pregnant women could protect infants.

It is recommended that pregnant women be vaccinated in

their third trimester, and that infants should receive the DTaP vaccination (diphtheria, tetanus toxoids, and acellular pertussis) vaccine as soon as possible, with the first dose recommended as early as six weeks.
California had also experienced an epidemic in 2010, when nearly 10,000 cases were reported. It was determined that the intentional refusal of vaccinations, as well as under-vaccinated individuals were highly likely to have contributed to recent and past pertussis outbreaks.

Prevalence of Cases Based on Geographical Location

Pertussis is not a geographically specific disease. It's found in the United States, Great Britain, the Middle East, Asia, South America, and in the Pacific, and everywhere in between.

Outbreaks in Iraq, Afghanistan, and the United States are only a few that have made news in recent months and years.

Data provided by the World Health Organization (WHO) in 2013 determined that over 135,000 cases of pertussis were reported around the world. In 2008, 195,000 died. Data regarding immunization coverage determined that approximately 129 countries around the world had achieved at least 90% immunization coverage (with DPT3 – 3 doses of Diphtheria, Pertussis, Tetanus vaccine) in infants as of 2013.

Latin America and the United States as well as a great portion of China, Russia, and Southeast Asia are also among the highest percentiles regarding immunization coverage.

Approximately 27 countries, including India, Pakistan and Africa, report between 50% and 80% coverage, while seven countries, found predominantly in Africa, provide less than 50%

immunization coverage.

The number of cases of pertussis reported since 1980 has been reduced drastically due to DTP3 coverage. A high number of cases of pertussis were found in the early 1980s, and as of 1990, they had decreased, with an average of less than 500,000 individuals affected by pertussis around the world.

Providing education regarding the benefits of immunizations is still a continual challenge for health providers around the globe. The focus of the World Health Organization (WHO) is on the monitoring and assessment of strategies that can reduce mortality as well as morbidity for vaccine preventable disease processes.

Regardless of the great strides made in this area, a variety of global health organizations including WHO, the CDC, and UNICEF, have been unable to completely eradicate pertussis or the mortality caused by it around the world.

In 2008 alone, nearly 195,000 children under five years of age died from what is considered a preventable disease today.

Pertussis is not the only disease that causes many deaths among young children around the world. Incidents of measles, mumps, polio, rubella, and tetanus are also prevalent, especially in India, Indonesia, Nigeria and the Russian Federation.

According to data provided by the World Health Organization, the greatest numbers of children who have died from pertussis come from African regions, although deaths still remain high in Indonesia (an alarming number of nearly 6,000 in 2005 alone), Iran, the Russian Federation, and India.

The World Health Organization launched their Global Vaccine Action Plan in 2011, with their goal to prevent "millions" of deaths by 2020. They aim to do this by providing greater access to existing vaccines around the world.

Promoting education regarding routine immunizations is the focus of WHO and other health organizations in order to reduce deaths in young children when it comes to vaccine-preventable diseases.

According to the strategic objectives of the Global Vaccine Action Plan, WHO wants to "Ensure that everyone everywhere receives the safest vaccines possible and that safety concerns are not a cause of hesitancy in using vaccines."

According to the CDC and other medical experts, the side effects from the whooping cough vaccine are extremely minimal, and are typically mild. The majority of children don't experience any side effects, while some might develop some redness, minimal swelling, and short-term discomfort from the shot itself at the injection site. Some may develop a low-grade fever and some may vomit.

Side effects typically occur in up to 1 out of every 4 children,

with most of the side effects being mild. We'll discuss the pros and cons of vaccinations in a later section.

Tetanus, diphtheria, and pertussis can be very serious, even for those who are in their adolescent years and adulthood. Why? Because tetanus, otherwise known as lockjaw, causes muscle tightening and stiffness all over the body, though it is most commonly identified by a painful tightening of the facial muscles, hence the nickname.

The condition can tighten the muscles in the neck and head to the extent that you cannot open your mouth or swallow. Tetanus, according to the CDC, kills approximately 1 out of every 10 people who are infected.

Diphtheria is a condition that causes a thick coating to form in the throat as well as the release of a toxin. If left untreated, it can lead to difficulty breathing, heart failure, paralysis, and sometimes, death.

Pertussis, or whooping cough, has already been described as a condition that causes moderate to severe coughing spells. This condition can cause difficulty breathing, and for some, the coughing spells can cause vomiting and sleep disruption.

About half of infants below 12 months who are diagnosed with pertussis are hospitalized. Complications experienced by infants include apnea, pneumonia, and less commonly, seizures and death.

Nearly 1 in every 100 adolescents and approximately 3 out of every 100 adults diagnosed with pertussis are hospitalized, and may experience some complications that can include pneumonia, weight loss, rib fractures (from heavy coughing), incontinence, and sometimes even death.

All three of these conditions are caused by bacteria. Pertussis and diphtheria are spread by sneezing or coughing. You can contract tetanus through scratches, cuts or other open wounds on the body that have typically come into contact with a rusty object such as a nail.

Before the advent of routine vaccines, nearly 200,000 cases every year of pertussis and diphtheria were noted in the United States. Since the advent of routine vaccinations, cases have ebbed.

Tetanus has also dropped by nearly 100%, and pertussis cases have decreased by approximately 80%.

Interestingly, as of 2013, a new strain of pertussis was noted, missing a formerly common component called pertactin, a protein that is found in the pertussis bacteria and gives it the ability to attach to the lining in the airways.

In a nutshell, acellular vaccines replaced whole-cell vaccines in numerous countries around the world (including the US, Australia and Western Europe).

However between 2008 and 2012, nearly 30% of pertussis outbreaks were believed to be caused due to the fact that the Bordetella pertussis isolates didn't express the vaccine antigen pertactin. This effectively made the newer vaccines, though with fewer side effects, less effective than the original vaccines created with whole cell pertussis.

In fact, recent studies have concluded that Bordetella pertussis isolates that do not express pertactin (PRN) are increasing in regions where acellular pertussis vaccines have been used for over 7 years.4
Medical experts agree that the pertussis vaccination in childhood provides protection for several years, but gradually wears off as the child ages. For this reason, increasing numbers of outbreaks are being seen in the world, as noted with the previous mention of the two outbreaks in California.

Improved technologies, relating to diagnosis and alterations in pertussis vaccines has not only made it easier to identify and diagnose pertussis, but in our approaches to vaccination. Primary among which is the new acellular pertussis vaccination as opposed to the whole cell pertussis vaccination, which was first introduced to the public in the 1990s.

According to the CDC, the vaccines continue to be effective in preventing and/or reducing the severity of pertussis. Before the widespread use of the vaccines, approximately 200,000 cases a year were noted in the United States, and those numbers have decreased drastically.

Note: It should also be understood that the new strain of pertussis (that's missing the protein pertactin) is not antibiotic resistant.
Antibiotics that are commonly recommended for the early treatment of pertussis continue to remain effective.

As a recap, pertussis was one of the major causes of childhood illness and disease as well as mortality in the 20th century. In the 21st century, and as of 2004, an estimated 300,000 children from around the world died of the disease.

Chapter Two: Causes

What causes pertussis? It should be noted that while doctors have identified the bacteria that causes the disease, they haven't determined where it comes from. It should also be noted that the pertussis bacteria does not have an animal or insect source. It's a strictly human disease.

It's not only important to know what pertussis is, but how it is transmitted. Because pertussis is a respiratory disease that is spread by respiratory droplets, it's also extremely contagious. Why? Because respiratory droplets can occur with sneezing and coughing.

When people are in close contact with an infected person who sneezes and breathes in the bacteria in the droplets, they can develop the disease. It should be noted that transmission caused by contact with contaminated articles occurs less frequently than someone who has, for example, been sneezed on.

As the Bordetella bacteria releases toxins into the upper respiratory system, the cilia become damaged, which in turn leads to swelling and inflammation.

Bordetella pertussis bacterium has this negative impact on the respiratory system through its production of toxins that inflame and literally paralyze portions of respiratory structures. Once the bacteria 'sticks' or makes its home in the epithelial cells of the lungs, the toxin prevents the cilia from functioning.

The job of the cilia is to clear mucus and other debris from the lungs. As the cilia are prevented from doing their job, the body's response is to cough, which helps to remove some of the build-up of mucus (and also spread the disease to others).

Let's break this down. The upper respiratory tract is composed of the nose, as well as the nostrils, the entire nasal cavity, the mouth, throat, and larynx.

Each of these components of the upper respiratory tract is lined with mucous membranes. These mucous membranes secrete mucus, which serves to trap small particles before they get deeper into the respiratory system (such as the lungs).

Small particles can range from anything like dust and cigarette smoke to pollen and other allergens. The cilia look like tiny hairs that line the surface of these mucous membranes, and are designed to transport or move the small particles that they capture up and out of the airways.

In fact, these little tiny hair-like cilia provide a very important function in protecting the entire respiratory system. As you inhale air, it's warmed, moistened, and literally cleansed by the cilia and vascular mucous membranes lining the nose.

Think about fields of long grass waving with the wind on the plains. The cilia are always in motion, much like an ocean current. They're very tiny and cannot be seen by the naked eye. At any rate, cilia are vital in maintaining the health of the respiratory system.

Cilia not only lie in the mucous membranes of the upper respiratory system, but are also found in the membranes that line the airways of the lungs, including the surface of the bronchi. They constantly trap and remove foreign particles, bacteria, viruses, as well as phlegm located in the lower respiratory tract (the lungs) upward and out of the body.

Scientists have even gone so far as to say that many lung diseases or lung problems are the result of cilia that have ceased to function properly.

So, in a nutshell, the cilia provide a literal one-way street for the removal of particles from the upper and main respiratory system - toward the nasal cavity, or for the cilia located in the lungs, they move these particles to the throat.

So basically, when your nose drips or you cough, producing phlegm or mucus, you can thank your cilia for working hard to keep you healthy.

If the cilia do not function properly, or become swollen or inflamed (such as by the pertussis bacteria) they are unable to move properly, and this can interfere with and compromise lung and overall health.

The pathogenesis, or process by which pertussis causes disease in the respiratory system, can be broken down thus: bacteria attach themselves to the cilia of the mucous membranes and respiratory cells and produce the toxins that paralyze them. This creates inflammation, which, quite simply, interferes with the ability of the lungs to function and clear secretions.

Then, substances created by the pertussis bacteria enable the bad guys to proliferate and resist defenses initiated by the body's immune system response. While lymphocytes that fight infection and bacteria may be produced, their ability to fight the bacteria is drastically impaired.

Here are some quick facts about pertussis that every parent should know:

a) Pertussis is milder in adolescents and adults than it is in infants and children.

b) A person may be infected with the pertussis bacteria and be asymptomatic, or not present with any symptoms. This would be more common in older individuals.

c) Even a person who has a mild case of pertussis is capable of transmitting the infection to others.

d) Older people are often a primary source of infection for children.

Pertussis is very contagious. Studies have shown that secondary attacks of pertussis among household members average approximately 80%.

An individual diagnosed with pertussis is most infectious during the first two weeks after initial onset of coughing (in most cases approximately 2 weeks or 14 days) as well as during the catarrhal period (more on the stages of the disease process in just a bit).
Signs and Symptoms

Whooping cough may start off with symptoms similar to a common cold. Mild cold-like symptoms such as stuffy nose, sore throat, a general feeling of malaise, and a mild cough may be obvious.

However, as the illness progresses, you may notice more severe fits of coughing, many of which end with a whooping or wheezing sound as the individual inhales air in between the coughs or at the end of a series of coughs.

Within two weeks of infection, the coughing may grow more severe and is particularly noticeable at night. Parents may also notice a clear, thick mucus discharge from the nose. A child/adolescent/adult may experience these bouts of coughing for up to two to three months.

Coughing may not become severe enough to be particularly noticeable until bouts of coughing seem to go on for quite a time, with up to 15 coughs at a time.

The particular sound of the coughs is also noticeable. These coughs are often followed by the sound of a high-pitched or deep and prolonged in-drawn breath that can also be equated with a whooping sound.

After the coughing attacks subside, breathing may return to normal, but in a short period of time, another coughing fit may follow.

The cough produced by pertussis may also be defined as 'loose' and is often accompanied by the presence of great globs of mucus. Young children typically end up swallowing that mucus, or you may notice bubbles appearing at the nose following a fit of coughing. For some, a gagging or vomiting reflex may also closely follow a fit of prolonged coughing.

Parents of very young children and infants should watch for difficulty breathing, as choking on the mucus as well as a pause in breathing known as apnea may occur. Apnea can be defined as a prolonged episode during which breathing may stop.
Note: a lack of oxygen or episodes of apnea will cause the skin to turn blue. This doesn't happen right away. Pay attention to your child's skin color. The first sign of lack of oxygen caused by apnea may include a bluish tinge noticed around the edges of the mouth and face. That noted, every parent should know how to provide first aid for apnea and/or call for an ambulance or any

other medical emergency service.

It's also important for parents to be aware that nearly one quarter of children diagnosed with whooping cough may develop pneumonia, which also causes difficulty breathing. We will also discuss preventative measures you can take to help reduce the risk of your child contracting pneumonia.

Another common symptom of pertussis is a condition that you may feel has nothing to do with the lungs, called otitis media, otherwise known as a middle ear infection. That's because the sinuses and the ear, and hence ear infections, are commonly linked to lung conditions that not only include pertussis, but allergies. The sinuses connect to the ear canals, so basically, any upper respiratory tract infection that is accompanied by coughing can affect the ears.

Otitis media is the medical term for an ear infection that commonly plagues infants and young children. The technical term applies to inflammation of the middle ear, and in this situation, an excess of fluid builds up in the middle ear.

Middle ear infections are relatively common when associated with allergies, exposure to environmental irritants, as well as upper respiratory viral infections. The middle ear is basically a space filled with air that is equalized with pressure outside the ears via the Eustachian tube. This tube connects the middle ear to the nasopharynx, which is the back part of the nose and throat.

In most cases, the ear pain (otalgia) experienced as a symptom with acute otitis media, resolves on its own. Parents should be aware that most cases of otitis media will not benefit from antibiotics.

In children too young to define what they're feeling, it's important for parents to watch for other signs and symptoms of middle ear infections. These can generally be noticed when an infant or child pulls on their ear or ears.

They may have difficulty balancing (the inner ear is associated with balance as well as hearing), or difficulty hearing. You may even notice a discharge draining from the ears. Otitis media often causes children to become cranky, irritable, and cry.

The CDC recommends that parents should always take steps to prevent ear infections by reducing their exposure to secondhand smoke, excessive air pollution, as well as keeping their children up to date with recommended immunizations. We'll be discussing more of the pros and cons regarding immunizations in a later section.

How Does Whooping Cough Progress?

Whooping cough generally runs its course in about six to eight weeks, though sometimes 12 weeks or even longer. The condition generally progresses through three different stages:

Catarrhal - This stage of the condition lasts approximately one to two weeks and is commonly accompanied by:

a)   Sneezing

b)   Nasal congestion

c)   A low-grade fever

d)   Mild cough

e) Tearing of the eyes

f) Runny nose (rhinorrhea)

g) Conjunctival suffusion

As you can see, the above description of symptoms sound like the common cold – which is why most don't seek or realize they need treatment until they get to the second stage, which is:

Paroxysmal – During this stage, episodes of coughing that last from one to three minutes is common, and can include five to fifteen coughs. Many of these coughing 'fits' are accompanied by the typical "whooping" sound associated with the illness. Your child may also become red in the face from the coughing episode, or gag or vomit following the episode. (This stage may last between one week and six weeks).

Convalescent - Following the first two stages of pertussis, you may notice that your child has a persistent cough that can last for many weeks.

In children, complications of whooping cough include pneumonia and apnea.

When it comes to adolescents and adults, complications such as urinary incontinence, difficulty sleeping, pneumonia, and rib fractures are relatively common. Rib fractures often occur due to severe bouts of coughing.

When to see the Doctor

Parents are the first to notice when a cough lasts longer or grows more severe and are typically quick to take their child to the pediatrician.

Doctors can diagnose whooping cough based on symptoms as well as through cultures of samples of mucus taken from the back of the throat or the nose which are used to confirm the diagnosis.

In most cases, children with pertussis will recover completely, although recovery can be slow. However, parents should be aware that a small percentage (approximately 1% to 2%) of children under the age of one, die from whooping cough.

The CDC statistics report that in the years between 2004 and 2008, approximately 111 deaths were reported in the United States. Children under three months of age accounted for approximately 83% of these deaths.

How is Pertussis Diagnosed?

Diagnosis of pertussis is made following a visit to the doctor and a thorough clinical history. For example, if a child or individual has a cough that lasts more than two weeks and is accompanied with the typical "whooping" sound, or post-cough vomiting.

These symptoms in addition to lab tests can provide a diagnosis of pertussis.

A few of the most common lab tests generally used to confirm pertussis include:

NP swab and culture. This is considered the "gold standard" test for diagnosing whooping cough. A swab is taken from the mucosal lining of the back of the nasopharynx, which is the section of the upper airway just behind the nose.

The specimen collected then undergoes a culture. It is transferred to a medium that encourages growth of the bacteria Bordetella pertussis.

If the swab has been taken from an individual with pertussis infection, then the culture should show growth. Cultures detect pertussis in 80% to 90%6 of cases during the catarrhal and early paroxysmal stages.

Direct fluorescent antibodies. If a person has been exposed to pertussis, this test detects antibodies that have been generated against the bacteria by the individual's immune system. However, this test is believed to have 'variable sensitivity and low specificity according to the National Institutes of Health.

Polymerase chain reaction (PCR).

This is a molecular test which detects DNA sequences of the bacterium Bordetella pertussis. The specimen which is tested is taken from a swab of the back of the nasal cavity.

Potential Complications of Pertussis

It's important to seek treatment if you or your child has been diagnosed with pertussis. The disease can lead to complications. Does this mean that you'll experience such complications? No. But some infants, children, adolescents, and adults do. You should be informed about such complications – just in case.

Potential complications as a result of pertussis or whooping cough may be present in certain individuals, especially when that person (adult, child, or infant) has another health issue, illness, disease, or medical condition.

One of the most common is called secondary bacterial pneumonia. Secondary bacterial pneumonia is a common cause of death in influenza epidemics, according to the US National Library of Medicine and National Institutes of Health.

Secondary bacterial pneumonia is also believed to be the leading cause of death in pertussis-related cases, occurring in approximately 17% of infants under the age of six months.

Additional complications involving the neurologic functions of the body are also possible, including seizures and encephalopathy (a disorder of the brain).

According to the article (Case 1: The deadly danger of Pertussis), nearly 2% of infants experience seizures, and approximately 0.4% develop encephalopathy.

In addition, severe bouts of coughing may cause hypoxia, or a drastic reduction in oxygen supply to the brain, which can contribute to such seizures.

It is also believed that the toxins produced by the pertussis bacterium may cause these neurologic complications, and it should be noted that most of these complications are observed in infants.

Additional complications, though less severe than those listed above, can include otitis media (middle ear infection), dehydration, and anorexia, due to the inability to eat because of the severe coughing fits and/or vomiting episodes that may follow.

A child who has become very ill due to whooping cough may be hospitalized due to breathing difficulties. Some of these children may need to be placed on mechanical ventilation systems based on their situation and scenario.

Older children with mild symptoms of the illness are generally treated at home, but parents should be aware that most cough medicines are not recommended, as they don't do much to relieve symptoms and often prevent coughing, the body's natural method of trying to relieve congestion and expel foreign bacteria.

Based on the severity of the disease and the age of the child, additional complications caused by extreme coughing, and the pressure effects of these coughing spasms, can include:

pneumothorax (puncture of chest wall leading to air in the chest cavity), subdural hematomas (bleeding around the brain), hernias (abnormal protrusions of organs), epistaxis (nose bleeds), and even rectal prolapse (when the rectum extends beyond the anus). While such complications are not common, they can occur.

A Few More Quick Facts about Pertussis

According to the CDC:

a)   As of 2012, nearly 50,000 cases of whooping cough were reported in the US alone, and yet hundreds if not thousands more can go unreported or incorrectly diagnosed. The number of cases of pertussis has gradually risen. Compare that to the number of cases in 1955, listed as nearly 63,000.

b)   Fits of coughing that are caused by the pertussis bacterium can last for up to 10 weeks in some children and young adults. For this reason, it may often be nicknamed "the 100 day cough".

c) The CDC recommends the DTaP vaccination for children and infants, and the Tdap for pre-teenagers, teens, and adults, reminding the public that efficacy of the vaccination fades over time.

d) An individual vaccinated with the pertussis vaccine can contract the disease, although in the great majority of such cases, the symptoms and the length of the disease is less severe.

e) As of 2012, nearly 16 million cases of pertussis were reported worldwide, causing approximately 195,000 deaths annually.

In 2013, nearly 29,000 cases of pertussis were reported, but as of mid-August 2014, the CDC had already received information that more than 17,000 cases had been reported, according to the Journal of Family Practice.

Recommendations were made by the doctors who wrote the journal article (Staying ahead of Pertussis), and members of the Family Medicine Residency Program, the Central Maine Medical Center, Lewiston; Department of Family Medicine, and the University of North Carolina at Chapel Hill. The practice recommendations include:

1) One-time Tdap (tetanus/diphtheria/acellular pertussis) vaccine for adults below the age of 64 who require a tetanus booster;

2) Suspect a case of pertussis in a patient who presents with an ongoing whooping cough for at least two weeks;

3) Prescribe a macrolide antibiotic for infants, children, and

adults with pertussis.

Indeed, the article states that even though the vaccination rate against pertussis is relatively high, it is still one of the only vaccine-preventable diseases that has shown a rise in recent cases.

It is strongly believed that the increase in cases seen today are as result of the pertussis vaccines' efficacy fading over time, coupled by increased awareness of the disease and its symptoms by doctors, therefore leading to more accurate reporting.

However, the article also warns that adults should not forget to get their vaccinations. The graphic below provides suggestions regarding adult pertussis vaccination based on the Journal of Family Practice.

Source: Journal of Family Practice - http://www.jfponline.com/specialty-focus/infectious- diseases/article/staying-ahead-of-pertussis.html

Chapter Three: Traditional Treatments

For children who have been exposed to pertussis, antibiotics such as erythromycin are recommended as a preventive measure.

However, timing is important in the treatment of pertussis with antimicrobials (another name for antibiotics), according to the CDC.
They are most effective when started early on in the course of the illness, within the first few weeks of developing symptoms.

Antibiotics may also be recommended in children for additional infections which may be associated with pertussis, including ear infections and pneumonia, although antibiotics are of little use in viral infections.

Erythromycin has long been the antibiotic drug of choice when treating pertussis. In most cases, it's very effective in eradicating the bacterial organisms from secretions.

In addition, erythromycin may help decrease the potency of the disease in a person's body, reducing communicability. In some cases, and when identified early, erythromycin may also actually modify progression of the illness.

Other antibiotics that have also been proven effective in the treatment of pertussis include:

a)   Azithromycin

b)   Trimethoprim-sulfamethoxazole

To date, doctors continue to recommend antibiotics to anyone who has come into close contact with someone who has been diagnosed with pertussis, regardless of their vaccination status or age.

Note: It is strongly recommended that parents do not self-diagnose their children. Because the early symptoms of pertussis can often mimic the common cold, allergies, rhinitis, or other upper respiratory tract conditions, it is best to schedule a visit a your local clinic or with your pediatrician.

Why did they stop using the Whole Cell Pertussis Vaccine?
The whole cell pertussis vaccine was developed in the mid-1930s, and by the 1940s was often combined and released as the DTP (diphtheria, tetanus, and pertussis) vaccine.

After the traditional three doses, immunization had an efficacy rate between 70% and 90% in individuals, with protection that lasted between five and 10 years. Reactions to the pertussis vaccine were relatively mild but were common, as well as a localized to the injection site.

The whole cell pertussis vaccine was considered successful in preventing more serious cases of pertussis, although it has only recently been understood that protection efficacy will decrease over time.

It should be noted that whole cell pertussis vaccinations are no longer being used in the United States, although they are still utilized in certain countries around the world.

The acellular pertussis vaccine has been used since the early

1990s. This vaccine is composed of sub-unit sized, inactive and purified components of the Bordetella pertussis cellular structure.

Due to advances in technology, these vaccines have also been developed to use for different age groups, utilizing different components in variable concentrations based on the age of the patient being given the vaccine.

Today, acellular pertussis vaccinations come only as a combination with diphtheria and tetanus toxoids.

The pediatric form for the pertussis vaccination (DTaP) is commonly used throughout the United States. Three of these formulations have been devised.
The DTaP vaccine is designed as a pediatric form of the vaccination and has been approved for children six weeks of age up to seven years of age.

The acellular pertussis vaccine used for adolescents and adults is known as Tdap. It is approved for individuals aged 10 to 64 (this version is known as Boosttix) while another, for the same age group, is known as Adacel).

Yes, the acronyms and the similarity between the DTaP and the Tdap can be confusing. We won't get into a deep description regarding the components of the toxoids, but it is important for parents to know exactly what's contained in these vaccinations in order to alleviate common questions or concerns.

After following questions posted by parents on online community boards, the reason that many parents give for not vaccinating their children, in recent years, is related with their concerns regarding side effects or the misinformation that the vaccines actually cause the disease. They don't.

Following is a review regarding the different compositions of the acellular pertussis vaccines.

One form of the vaccine is known as Infanrix (GlaxoSmithKline) - composed of three pertussis antigens, including inactivated pertussis toxin (PT), pertactin and filamentous hemagglutinin FHA.

Tripedia (sanofi pasteur) - composed of two pertussis components (FHA and PT) in equalized amounts (supply of this vaccine has now been discontinued in the US).

Daptacel (sanofi pasteur) - composed of five pertussis components (PT, pertactin, FHA, and types II and III of fimbriae)

All three of these above-mentioned vaccines are given in a single dose vial or syringe.

Pertussis Vaccine for Adolescents and Adults

Acellular pertussis vaccines for adolescents and adults (Tdap) were first licensed in the United States in 2005 and readily available to the public in 2006.

Two vaccinations of this type are available and both are combined with tetanus toxoids as well as a small amount of diphtheria toxoid – different from those of the pediatric doses. These vaccines are also given in single-dose syringes or vials.

It should be noted that clinical trials regarding the efficacy of DTaP vaccinations have been conducted around the world with a variety of the specific products listed above (Infanrix, Tripedia, Daptacel).

Such clinical trials have been ongoing since the early 1990s, not only in the United States, but in Europe and Africa. Efficacy ratings ranging from 80% to 85% for the vaccines that are currently licensed for use in the United States have been documented.

In Sweden, the product Daptacel is rated at approximately 85% efficacy, while in Germany, Tripedia ranks at 80%, and in Italy, Infanrix ranks at approximately 84%.

Side effects of the newer acellular pertussis vaccinations are fewer than those that were noted in the earlier version of the vaccine (the whole cell DTP).

Most health organizations throughout the world provide a routine and suggested DTaP primary vaccination schedule.

Dose	Age	Minimum interval
Primary 1	2 months	---
Primary 2	4 months	4 weeks
Primary 3	6 months	4 weeks
Primary 4	15 to 18 months	6 months

The fourth dose is typically offered between 6 to 12 months after the third dose in order to maintain an adequate level of immunity for the preschool-aged child.

In most cases, the fourth dose should be administered between 15 and 18 months of age, although when using Daptacel, the dose should be given between 17 and 20 months.

Your pediatrician will know the vaccination schedule based on the specific brand or component of the vaccination they're using.

So, in regard to the fourth dose typically being recommended between 15 and 18 months of age it can be given earlier if:

a) the child is 12 months of age, and it has been 6 months since their third dose, and

b) they are unlikely to return for another visit at 15 to 18 months of age.

It is also recommended that any child who receives all the doses before their fourth birthday should also receive a fifth booster shot or dose of the DTaP before entering school.

However, the booster dose is not necessary, but still may be given, if the fourth dose of the original and primary series of vaccinations were given on or after the fourth birthday.

The booster shot effectively increases the levels of antibodies and decreases the risk of school-age children having the potential to transmit the disease to younger children in the household or at school among those who have not been completely vaccinated.

It should also be noted that if the vaccinations are not given directly based on the schedule, or if a delay occurs, this does not reduce the immunity level that has been reached by completing the entire primary series.

It is not necessary to restart the entire series of doses regardless of the time frame that has passed between doses. For example, if you are late or delayed in getting a third dose on schedule, your pediatrician will not recommend that you restart the entire series, but will simply give that third dose at that time.

Parents should also note that the Food and Drug Administration in the United States has approved both Tdap vaccinations (Boostrix and Adacel) for individuals who have already completed their recommended childhood vaccination series.

Medical experts are now recommending that children between the ages of 11 and 18 get another booster shot, and that individuals between the ages of 19 and 64 undergo another series of the Dtap vaccination series in order to restore adequate levels of immunity that may have faded over time.

Note: In recent years, it has also been recommended that any person over 65 years of age who is expected to or who will likely come into contact with unvaccinated children under the age of 12 months, be re-vaccinated with a Tdap vaccine. This is also something for parents to think about. Aging parents and grandparents who may have been exposed to or are even carrying the pertussis bacteria may come into contact with your child, so better to be safe than sorry.

If you are pregnant, and have not received a Tdap vaccination, it is recommended that you do so, preferably during either the late second trimester or the third trimester (after approximately 20 weeks gestation).

For women who are not given the Tdap vaccination during pregnancy, it is highly recommended that they get one immediately post-partum (after birth).

Along those lines, any adolescent, adult, child care provider, siblings, grandparents, or others who will be in and out, and have close contact with your infant, should also be open to receiving a single dose of Tdap in order to reduce the risk of pertussis transmission.

When should this happen? The CDC recommends at least two weeks before any contact with the infant.

More about Pediatric Pertussis Vaccines

Let's talk about Pediarix (GlaxoSmithKline), approved by the FDA in 2002. This contains five components and is a combination vaccine of:

a) DTaP (Infanrix)

b) Hepatitis B (Engerix-B)

c) Inactivated polio vaccine

This vaccine is recommended at approximately 6 weeks of age. It's approved for three doses at two months, four months, and six months of age, but is not recommended as a booster dose.

This combination vaccine has been licensed for children between the ages of six weeks and six years of age. It can be used interchangeably with another pertussis containing vaccine.

Pentacel is also a combination vaccine. It contains lyophilized Hib (ActHIB) that has been modified with a liquid solution containing DTaP and IPV (inactivated polio virus vaccine).

Doses of this vaccine are recommended for children between six weeks of age through four years of age in four doses. This combination vaccine was approved and licensed by the Food and Drug Administration in the United States in mid-2008.

The Kinrix combined vaccination contains DTaP and inactivated polio virus vaccine. Approved in 2008 by the Food and Drug Administration in the United States, it's produced by GlaxoSmithKline.

This combination vaccine is only licensed for a fifth dose of DTaP or a fourth dose of IPV in children between the ages of four and six under certain circumstances, and depending on the type or brand of their first three doses of the pertussis vaccination. Note: In children who have been diagnosed with neurologic disorders (cerebral palsy, developmental delay, controlled idiopathic epilepsy, etc.), recommendations are either to delay and assess the situation, or to vaccinate.

For example, doctors are recommended to delay and assess children with underlying conditions such as prior seizure history, a suspected or diagnosed neurological disorder, or any neurological event that occurs between doses.

In the cases where the child is classified as stable or the neurologic condition has resolved, the recommendation is to vaccinate.

In cases where there is a family history of neurologic disease, seizures, or conditions that are stable and resolved, they are not contraindications to obtaining a pertussis vaccine. In other words, vaccines can be given in these circumstances.

Chapter Four: Pros and Cons of Vaccinations

History's Lessons – FAQs

Let's talk a moment about the actual science involved in vaccination research and testing. This is something that every parent needs to know. It's not enough to listen to the opinion of friends or even strangers, because this is your child. What if they're wrong? What if they're uninformed, or rely on myths rather than scientific fact?

Again, we're not trying to sway parents one way or another to vaccinate or not to vaccinate – what we are emphasizing is to be an informed parent.

Did you know that it can take between 10 and 15 years of research and study before any kind of vaccine is made available to the public?

The process is extremely detailed, involved, and extensive, and even the first exploration into the process can take several years of laboratory research and data collection. The first step that researchers take is to identify an antigen that can be used to actually inhibit or prevent disease processes.

At its most basic definition, an antigen is defined as a protein or carbohydrate substance such as a toxin or an enzyme that is capable of stimulating an immune response. Keep in mind that this is only the first step.

After years of research and development, in the United States for example, any test vaccine must be accepted and "cleared" by the United States Food and Drug Administration, and undergo at least three additional phases of clinical trials before they are ready for public dissemination.

These trials are broken into three separate and consecutive clinical trials performed on volunteers to test the efficacy of vaccines, as well as to determine the most appropriate and effective dosages.

These individuals are also observed for any signs of adverse side effects and so forth. These phases of vaccine testing and development can take another several years.

The last step before any vaccine is made available to the general public is composed of a Phase III clinical trial that can include up to tens of thousands of volunteers known as test groups.

These groups undergo careful testing and observation. Consider the fact that most medicines in the US, while also undergoing extensive testing and scrutiny, are used in patients and/or groups that are up to three times smaller than the clinical trial test subject groups required for vaccination testing.

However, even the conclusion of the three clinical trial phases is not the end of the process. Once the three phases of clinical trials have been completed and determined safe and ready for approval, the Food and Drug Administration will continue to follow and monitor the efficacy and safety of the vaccine. For example, numerous and different batches of the vaccine are tested. The same applies to any production processes as well as the facilities involved in the process of development of the vaccinations.

The Food and Drug Administration also carefully observes and monitors any reactions to the vaccinations. At this stage of the process, a number of state, province, and federal agencies may work together to not only collect, but track and analyze the data to ensure that the vaccinations are, and will continue, to remain safe for use by the general population.

For parents interested in learning more about this process, we suggest that you visit the website of the Centers for Disease Control and Prevention (CDC) and visit the Immunization Safety Office online.

Now you can see why the development of a vaccination can take between 10 to 15 years on average. You may wonder about that when you hear about seasonal flu vaccines provided by the US Food and Drug Administration, which are typically developed every year.
However, it's important to understand that it's not a vaccination itself that changes, but the antigen, especially when it comes to your yearly flu vaccine. The process of manufacturing a vaccination remains the same.

Unlike flu vaccines, which require scientists and researchers to "guesstimate" the type of flu virus that will be most prevalent during the forthcoming flu season, the process in creating stable vaccines such as those for pertussis, and other conditions remain the same.

A Brief Discourse on Disagreements Regarding School Requirements to Vaccination Prior to Admission

In the United States, a Pertussis vaccination is recommended for school-aged children, from preschool through college. For example, in California, the California Health and Safety Code,

(Sections 120325-120375) state: under these statutes, children in California are required to receive certain immunizations in order to attend public and private elementary and secondary schools, child care centers, family day care homes, nursery schools, day nurseries, and developmental centers.

Schools, child care centers, and family child care homes are required to enforce immunization requirements, maintain immunization records of all children in rolled, and submit reports.

Indeed, in addition to California, most state laws and school admission requirements recommend that students between the ages of four and six years require the following immunization schedule:

a) Diphtheria, tetanus, and pertussis (DTaP, DTP, or DT) - five doses (four doses is okay if one was given on or after fourth birthday)

b) Polio (OPV or IPV) – 4 doses (three doses is okay if one was given on or after fourth birthday)

c) Hepatitis B - three doses

d) Measles, mumps, and rubella (MMR) - two doses (both given on or after first birthday)

e) Varicella (chickenpox) - one dose

In states throughout the United States, parents must be able to show proof of their child's immunization record, and similar requirements also apply to students in transitional kindergarten environments.

In addition to the requirements for younger children, students entering school between the ages of 7 and 17 years are required to have the following immunizations:

a)   Diphtheria, tetanus, and pertussis (Dtap. DTP, DT, Tdap, or Td) - three doses (four doses required if last one was given before second birthday)

b)   Polio (OPV or IPV) - four doses (three doses okay if one was given on or after a second birthday)

c)   Measles, mumps, and rubella (MMR) - one dose (two doses required at seventh grade)

d)   Varicella (chickenpox) – admission of students between 7 to 12 years of age need one dose; for children between 13 and 17 years of age, two doses is required)

e)   Tetanus, diphtheria, and Pertussis – (Tdap) - one dose at seventh grade or for out of the state transfer admissions, at 8th grade through to 12th grade. One dose on or after the seventh birthday.

Depending on attitudes regarding immunization, which applies not only to California, but all states throughout the United States and in other countries, parents often are confused between the terminology of "required" versus "recommended" immunizations.

Keep in mind however, that while not all vaccines are absolutely required by state laws or regulations for school attendance, they are strongly recommended in order to protect the public.
In California (we will continue using this state as an example), state law requires that children receive specified immunizations

to not only protect themselves, but others who may come in contact with them, from a variety of childhood diseases.

In the United States, recommendations for the immunization schedules are developed by the American Academy of Pediatrics (AAP), the American Academy of Family Physicians (AAFP) and the Federal Advisory Committee on Immunization Practices (ACIP).

Numerous programs throughout the United States and other developed countries provide vaccinations for eligible children free of charge if parents cannot afford the vaccines, or if their health insurance does not cover them.

Local health departments are another option for low-cost and sometimes free vaccinations. Last but not least, local pharmacies and pharmacists may also provide Tdap vaccines and other types of vaccines for a very small fee.

What about Exemptions?

Exemptions for standardized and legal requirements for immunizations that are based on personal beliefs are known as a personal belief exemption. Such laws only recently came into effect in the United States.

Still using California as an example, and effective on January 1, 2014, a parent who wishes to exempt their child or children from one or even more of the required immunizations due to personal beliefs must provide the school, the child care facility, or the state caregiver, with a number of documents. The documents should include:

A statement signed by the parent as well as they child's health

care provider reiterating that the health care provider has provided the parent or parents with the information regarding the benefits as well as the risks of immunizations and the risks of contracting a vaccine-preventable disease.
A letter or affidavit requesting the exemption to one or more immunization because they are contrary to their beliefs.

A great majority of children whose parents have filed for certain exemptions do receive some of the recommended and required vaccinations – just not all of them.

Information regarding which vaccines their child or children have received should be indicated to the school or child care facility so that they are aware of which children have been or have not been vaccinated for vaccine-preventable disease processes, in order to help avoid spreading these diseases in a school environment.

However, not just anybody can sign the documentation to refuse immunizations based on personal beliefs. Only a certain number of healthcare providers or practitioners can sign the exemption form, and they must be licensed and credentialed in their state, province, or region. In California, these practitioners are limited to:

a) Medical doctor (MD)

b) Nurse practitioner (NP) who is authorized to offer or provide drugs

c) Doctor of osteopathic medicine (DO)

d) Physician Assistant (PA) who is authorized to provide and administer medications

e)   Naturopath doctor who is authorized to either order, furnish, provide, or administer medications or drugs under the supervision of a surgeon or a physician

f)   Credentialed school nurse (credentials are based on state, region, province, or country requirements)

The forms requesting exemption from one or more immunization are required to be delivered to the school facility, child care facility, or caregivers prior to admissions.

It's important for parents to research this timeframe based on their state, province, or region. Most forms are not accepted later than six months before the first day of school, entrance into a childcare facility, and so forth.

Exemptions based on religious practice are also allowed, especially in cases where the parents' religion does not permit medical treatment from healthcare providers or practitioners. In the United States, using religion as a basis against immunization is relatively common, even when parents do not practice a particular faith.

A newspaper article printed in 2007 mentioned that there are an increasing number of parents in the United States who are doing just that; claiming religious exemption to avoid having to vaccinate their children when their real rationale was either concerns about illness caused by the vaccines or skepticism over the efficacy of the vaccinations.

We'll discuss in more detail a few reasons why some parents are hesitant to vaccinate their children, including the belief that immunizations can cause autism. In fact, Dr. Paul Offit, former head of Infectious Diseases at Children's Hospital in

Philadelphia stated that such "default" exemptions and parents' resistance to immunizations and vaccines were nothing more than "an irrational, fear-based decision."In 2007, the number of exemptions, in percentage terms, numbered just several thousand among 3.7 million children, but those numbers are increasing.

Dr. Lance Rodewald, Director of the Centers for Disease Control's immunization services division, stated "

...when you choose not to get a vaccine, you're not just making a choice for yourself, you're making a choice for the person sitting next to you."

There will always be a pro and con, for and against, when it comes to vaccines and immunizations.
In the United States, approximately 28 states allowed parents to claim exemptions for religious or medical reasons only, but that was back in 2007. Twenty other states also allowed parents to specify philosophical or personal reasons, while a few states continue to only allow such exemptions based on medical reasons.

From 2003 to 2007, "religious" exemptions for kindergarten-aged students either doubled or tripled in the states that allowed only religious or medical exemptions.

Following are just a few additional statistics regarding the number of exemptions requested between the mid-1990s and 200614:
a) In Massachusetts between 1996 and 2006, the number of exemptions doubled from a 0.24% to 0.60%.

b) In Florida, the number of exemptions based on religious

claims rose from 661 in 2002 to 1249 in 2006, an increase of 0.3% to 0.6% for that state's student population. Other states, including New Hampshire, Alabama, and Georgia, also saw the rate of exemptions double.

c) Today, more parents apply for exemptions based on philosophical reasons than medical or religious reasons.

To Vaccinate or Not (Side Effects vs. Benefits) – FAQs about Vaccination

One of the standing arguments against vaccinations made by parents is that they don't believe that the vaccine is effective anyway, so why put their children through the pain of a shot?

First, let's state that children are a lot more resilient than we give them credit for. In regard to this argument, we broach this question: is the temporary ache or pain of a needle injection to be weighed against the potential (and painful) side effects of childhood diseases?

It is true that some parents belonging to specific resolutions such as Christian Scientists do have a history of authentic religious objection to most forms of modern medicine including blood transfusions, many forms of surgery, and so forth.

However, for others, it's a matter of distrust. Here are some of the most common reasons and beliefs that lead parents to choose not to immunize their children:

a) They're not convinced the vaccinations help

b) The vaccinations can make their children sick

c) The vaccinations can cause autism

d) Opinions are based on older vaccines that used to contain mercury-based preservatives, albeit in minimal amounts. Still, some continue to believe that the ingredients in pertussis and other childhood preventable disease vaccinations contribute to neurological disorders.

Now let's take a look at the pro-vaccine side. It is a reality that an unvaccinated child can contract the disease and even spread it to someone else who has not taken their vaccinations, or even those who have been vaccinated but are susceptible to milder forms of the disease.

As an example, again, referring to the article in USA Today15, an Indiana girl who had not been immunized contracted measles at an orphanage in 2005 and then returned to her church group. Within four weeks, 31 additional members of the church group contracted measles, which at that time, in 2005, was one of the nation's worst outbreaks of measles in over a decade.

One parent even stated, "I felt that the risk of the vaccine was worse than the risk of the actual disease."

Medical experts will emphasize that the risks of contracting pertussis are definitely more severe than mild side effects experienced by having the vaccine. More on that later.

The US Department of Health and Human Services (HHS) and the Health Resources and Services Administration (HRSA) enacted into law the National Childhood Vaccine Injury Act of 1986, created by the National Vaccine Injury Compensation Program (VICP).

This organization was first established in the 1980s not only to ensure and stabilize the cost of vaccines, but the supply of vaccines, as well as to provide individuals who claimed that the vaccinations caused injury and/or illness with the resources for information and compensation. The National Vaccine Injury Compensation Program is run by three federal government agencies in the US:

1) The US Department of Health and Human Services

2) The US Department of Justice

3) The US Court of Federal claims

A report brief dated from August 2011 and released by the Institute of Medicine of the National Academies documented adverse effects of vaccines regarding evidence and causality. The paper in essence stated that while vaccines cannot be guaranteed free from adverse effects or side effects, the great majority of those are extremely mild or very rare.

The paper emphasizes that in many cases, an adverse health problem following such a vaccination is due either to a coincidence or other health issues.

Researchers assessed a variety of data and evidence to determine whether adverse effects that did follow such vaccinations are specifically linked to vaccines, and if they were, they would be referred to in the paper as an adverse effect. For this reason, the National Childhood Vaccine Injury Act of 1986, again known as the National Vaccine Injury Compensation Program, was established by Congress in order to provide some sort of compensation to those claiming to have been injured by vaccinations.

In this paper, eight (8) common childhood vaccinations were studied:

1)   Varicella zoster vaccine (chickenpox)

2)   Influenza vaccines (not including the H1N1 influenza vaccine of 2009)

3)   Hepatitis B vaccine

4)   Human papillomavirus (HPV) vaccine

5)   Measles, mumps, and rubella (MMR) vaccine

6)   Hepatitis A vaccine

7)   Meningococcal vaccines

8)   Tetanus containing vaccines that do not carry whole cell pertussis components

The purpose of this paper was not to reassess the effectiveness or benefits of vaccines, but only to determine the risk of specifically defined "adverse events." For those who wish to read this report,

access the link provided in the footnote below16. However, to summarize, the evidence "favored" a rejection of a casual relationship between the following:

a)   MMR vaccine and autism

b)   MMR and Type 1 diabetes

c)   Dtap (tetanus) vaccine and Type 1 diabetes

d)   Inactivated influenza vaccine and Bell's Palsy (facial nerve weakness)

e)   Inactivated influenza vaccine and exacerbation of asthma or reactive airway disease episodes in children and adults

The data determined that there could be a "convincingly" supportive argument of a casual relationship between vaccinations that carried live vaccine such as Varicella zoster, and adverse reactions.

According to the study, vaccines may produce four specifically identified adverse reactions due to the virus strain they contain, including:

a)   Disseminated Varicella infection (widespread chickenpox rash
shortly after vaccination)

b)   Disseminated Varicella infection with subsequent infection resulting in pneumonia, meningitis, or hepatitis in individuals with demonstrated immunodeficiencies

c)   Vaccine strain viral reactivation (appearance of chickenpox rash months to years after vaccination)

d)   Vaccine strain viral reactivation with subsequent infection resulting in meningitis or encephalitis (inflammation of the brain).

As a result of the study, it was determined that individuals with somewhat compromised immune systems may be susceptible to adverse and somewhat rare effects from immunizations.

The conclusion of the study did determine that "certain characteristics" of individuals could place them at an increased risk of experiencing adverse effects, especially those with severe immunodeficiency. Such individuals may be adversely affected by vaccines that contain live viruses such as the Varicella and/or the measles, mumps, and rubella (MMR) vaccine.

The measles, mumps, and rubella vaccine (MMR) was also shown to have a supporting and casual relationship for two specific "adverse" events that included fainting, deltoid bursitis, syncope, some shoulder pain, and loss of motion. In essence, a casual relationship of adverse effects was found between:

a)   HPV vaccine and anaphylaxis (severe allergic reaction)
b)   MMR vaccine and temporary joint pain in female adults
c)   MMR vaccine and transient or temporary arthralgia (joint pain) in children

There has not been, to date, any scientifically documented or widespread cases that definitively link the side effects of the pertussis vaccination to serious issues.

HealthyChildren.org states that a number of side effects have long been blamed on the vaccinations, but proving this is extremely difficult. In a variety of cases, children do develop illness at some point after a vaccination is given, and parents are often quick to blame the immunization, though the specific evidence to support cause-and-effect association with immunizations or vaccines is just not available.

Let's explore a little deeper some of the most common myths that prevent parents from seeking immunizations or vaccines for their children.

DPT causes SIDS (Sudden Infant Death Syndrome)

Sudden Infant Death Syndrome (SIDS) is classified as one of the leading causes of death for infants between one month of age and one year of age, but is most common between the first and fourth months.

However, the major reason for SIDS has been determined as being related to babies who are used to sleeping on their backs but are then (for various reasons) placed on their tummies to sleep.
This is common in situations where a family member or someone else places the infant to sleep on their bellies, which results in a semi-medical term known as unaccustomed tummy sleeping. This can increase the risk of SIDS in some babies, especially those who are already used to sleeping on their backs.

SIDS is not caused by immunizations, choking, or vomiting. Let's explain further. Typically, the first diphtheria, tetanus and pertussis (DTP vaccine) is delivered in babies at approximately two months of age, which is coincidentally, the time in their young lives that they are at the highest risk of SIDS.
Researchers have engaged numerous studies dating back to the early 1980s to explore the perceived link between SIDS deaths and DTP vaccines. There is no scientific evidence linking the two, and research determined that the deaths of infants who had received the vaccine and those who didn't were fairly consistent with historical data of the highest rate of SIDS deaths occurring between one and four months of age.

MMR Vaccine causes Autism

As mentioned earlier, it has often been suggested by parents that the MMR vaccine is linked to autism. Autism is classified under an umbrella of severe and chronic developmental disorders typically diagnosed in young toddlers or young children.

In 2001 and 2004, the Institute of Medicine Immunization Safety Review Committee, an independent organization which had no interest in pharmaceuticals or governmental recommendations on vaccines, assessed and studied the potential link between autism and the MMR vaccine (eight times) and found no evidence to support this belief.

The American Association of Physicians, conducted a study, and they also came to the same conclusion.

Vaccines cause mercury poisoning

Let's talk about the risk of mercury poisoning. Starting in the 1930s, one of the ingredients in some of the vaccines provided to children contained a component called thimerosal, a preservative that contained mercury. This preservative was added to the vaccines because it enhanced prevention of bacterial or fungal contamination.

However, the Institute of Medicine Immunization Safety Review Committee studied the link between the vaccines that contained thimerosal and developmental or neurologic disorders, which ranged from speech and language delays, attention deficit hyperactivity disorder (ADHD) as well as autism. They rejected any type of a casual relationship between them.

As of 2001, vaccines are available that do not contain this preservative, and indeed, some vaccines, contrary to popular belief (including the chickenpox, polio, and MMR vaccines), never contained this preservative.

Additional myths regarding immunizations and their link to a variety of immune disorders, including Type 1 diabetes, asthma, and even multiple sclerosis, have been studied by the Institute of Medicine Immunization Safety Review Committee. No specific cause-and-effect relationships have been determined between any of the vaccinations and immune disorders, or the belief that Hepatitis B vaccines can cause Multiple Sclerosis, Guillain-Barre Syndrome or numerous other types of nervous system disorders.

The source for this information is "Immunizations and Infectious Diseases: an Informed Parents Guide, the American Academy of Pediatrics, 2006", and can be found on the HealthyChildren.org website from the American Academy of Pediatrics.

Parents are encouraged to inform themselves about vaccines and not to rely on innuendo, myth, or uninformed opinions of others. It has been established that yes, some children and even adults may be susceptible to some side effects or adverse events, but in most cases, these are limited to those who have some type of immunological dysfunction, and are limited to the immunizations or vaccines that contain live viral agents.

Vaccine Reactions

The reactions that an infant, child, adolescent, or adult may experience following a pertussis vaccine may differ. Again, while there is a chance of reaction in anybody who receives a vaccination, just as there are risks for those obtaining even minor surgical procedures, the side effects and risks are typically mild.

Here are a few of the more common reactions to Tdap vaccines as defined by the CDC:

Mild Symptoms (classified as those that do not typically appear with any activities)

a) Temporary pain where the shot was given (approximately 3 in every 4 adolescents and 2 in every 3 adults experience mild discomfort).

b) Redness or swelling at the location of the shot (approximately 1 in every 5 people experience this side effect).

c) Mild fever (approximately 100.4°F or 38°C) - approximately 1 in every 25 adolescents or 1 in every 100 adults experience a mild fever.

d) Headache (roughly 3 or 4 people in every 10).

e) Weariness (approximately 1 person out of every 3 or 4).

f) Stomachache, nausea, vomiting, or diarrhea (approximately 1 in every 10 adults and approximately 1 in every 4 adolescents).

g) Generalized body aches, sore joints, chills, rash, and though uncommon, swollen glands.

Moderate Symptoms (do not require medical attention but may interfere with some activities)

a) Pain at the shot location (approximately 1 in 5 adolescents or one in 100 adults).

b) Redness or swelling at location (approximately 1 in every 16 adolescents and 1in every 25 adults).

c) Fever above 102°F or 39°C (approximately 1 in every 100

adolescents or 1 in every 250 adults).

d)   Headaches (approximately 3 in every 20 adolescents or 1 in every 10 adults).

e)   Stomach ache, nausea, vomiting, or diarrhea (approximately 1 to 3 people in every 100).

f)   Swelling of the entire arm (approximately 3 in every 100).

Mild and moderate side effects or reactions to the Tdap vaccine are temporary in nature, and most recover within a day or two. However, some severe problems can occur, and require medical attention.

Though rare, parents should watch for severe reactions which can include anaphylaxis. This is a severe allergic reaction that can occur after any kind of vaccine. However, this type of reaction occurs in less than one individual per million doses.

For a serious allergic reaction, you will notice:

a)   Swelling in the face and throat area

b)   Hives (skin rashes)

c)   Difficulty breathing

d)   Dizziness, weakness, and a racing pulse.

These symptoms can occur anywhere from a few minutes following the vaccination to several hours later. Parents are encouraged to watch their children for any signs of reaction or high fevers

If you do believe that your child, an adolescent or an adult is experiencing anaphylaxis, call your local emergency first responders, or take the individual to the nearest emergency room.

Who Should Not Get the Tdap Vaccine?

The CDC recommends that some people do not get the tetanus, diphtheria, and pertussis vaccine. This includes anyone who has had any type of severe allergic reaction to any of the components of the vaccine. Before you get vaccinated, inform your doctor if you have any severe allergies.

In addition, anyone who experienced seizures or even a coma within one week after receiving a childhood dose of the DTP or DTaP vaccine should not have the Tdap vaccine, although you should talk to your doctor about getting the tetanus and diphtheria portion of the vaccine. In addition, discuss the following with your doctor:

a) If you are not feeling good on the day of the shot.

b) Whether you have ever had Guillain-Barré Syndrome (an acute neurological condition where you experience progressive weakness).

c) If you have ever experienced severe swelling or pain following any vaccine that contained the tetanus, pertussis, or diphtheria components, or have epilepsy or another type of nervous system disorder.

What about Maternal Vaccination?

Maternal vaccination implies situations where a pregnant woman receives the vaccination in order to help protect the infant from the moment of birth until the infant reaches an age where active vaccination may be possible.

According to the US National Library of Medicine and the National Institutes of Health, maternal vaccination using whole cell pertussis vaccines do not create serious or adverse side effects in the mother or the child.

In one study, it was determined that maternal vaccination provides viable protection for newborn infants. Supporting documentation verifies the efficacy of maternal vaccination when it comes to protecting very young infants against pertussis.

The Journal article titled, "The case for maternal vaccination against pertussis (Lancet Infectious Diseases 200722) states that such vaccinations can be considered effective in decreasing both morbidity as well as mortality in newborn babies.

About those Scary Ingredients

That being said, there is plenty of controversy and disagreement when it comes to arguments against vaccinations. Again, one of the main reasons that parents have been against vaccinations is that they have "scary ingredients".

Vaccinations contain parts of a virus or bacteria germ. It's called an antigen. However, antigens have already been crippled, or otherwise disabled or killed before they're used to make the vaccine, so it cannot make people sick.

In many cases, an antigen is a substance, most often a protein that helps to stimulate the body in creating and producing an immune response so that it can protect itself against the risk from exposure to an actual disease.

Vaccines often contain additional ingredients that make them last longer, become more effective, and safer. A number of additives, residuals, or adjuvants (a component in many vaccines that enhance their ability to protect against the infection) may be involved in the production of the vaccine. These 'residuals' will be discussed in more detail in just a moment.

While today's vaccines do contain antigens, they contain far fewer antigens than in the past due to advancements in technology and biomedical sciences.

In addition, you should note that your child's body is very well designed (and equipped) to handle a variety of antigens presented at the same time. In fact, healthy babies are able to deal with multiple vaccinations because many of the antigens that are contained in those vaccinations are specifically designed for a baby's immune system. The truth of the matter is that a human baby is capable of "handling" quite a few more antigens than those found in your typical vaccine.

We will briefly mention, and will mention it again in a moment, the fact that many parents are concerned regarding the presence of thimerosal, or ethylmercury. These are organic forms of mercury that help to prevent contamination of vaccines.

However, it's important to note that this form of mercury is not the same as the type of mercury (methylmercury) that has the potential, in specific amounts, to damage the central nervous system. All routine vaccines required to childhood are now produced essentially free of thimerosal, including flu vaccines.

Making the Decision

The bottom line is that every parent must determine the safety and efficacy of vaccines on their own. It's a personal decision. It's easy to rely on word-of-mouth or to be swayed by one argument against another. However, it's important to be able to separate myth from fact when it comes to vaccines. Rely on facts and scientific research when making a decision regarding vaccinations.

For some reason, great majorities of people are skeptical about scientific research as well as data and analysis, statistics and other information provided by government agencies or medical facilities. But at the same time, we trust ourselves, our spouses, and our children regarding the latest developments in medical technology, techniques, and procedures.

Know your child. Be aware if they seem to have a weakened immune system. If you are concerned about adverse reactions prior to receiving vaccinations for pertussis, have your pediatrician perform a thorough exam on your child to determine his or her overall health and wellness.

Yes, vaccinations, as well as a number of medications and drugs on the market today, can initiate adverse effects in individuals with a compromised immune system, or with other contributing health conditions. That goes for over-the-counter medications as well.

The majority of children do just fine with vaccines, but it's up to you, the parent, to weigh the pros and cons. We'll talk more about this in a little while. Your decision to immunize should be based on facts. To date, there has been no reliable and validated, scientific proof that vaccines cause any number of diseases or conditions, while at the other end of the spectrum, you can access literally hundreds of clinical studies and research that prove that vaccines do save lives, and have not been associated or otherwise linked to long-term side effects.

Over the past few decades, vaccinations have helped eradicate, or have come close to doing so, a number of preventable childhood diseases such as smallpox, which literally decimated entire communities prior to the advent of vaccinations. The same holds true for measles as well as pertussis.

Remember that your choice not to immunize does not only involve you and your child or immediate family members, but others too. Do your homework regarding recent outbreaks of preventable and sometimes life-threatening diseases that have occurred in society in recent years. We're not just talking about third world countries, but advanced societies. Why? Because people are no longer vaccinating, or they are delaying vaccinations.

Case in point - an 11-year-old boy who traveled from England in 2009 to a summer camp in New York spread the mumps virus to his fellow campers.

When it was all said and done, over 300 people had been infected within a year due to be an initial outbreak, but secondary outbreaks of the mumps disease eventually spread to Brooklyn, New York, Orange County, located in upstate New York, as well as New Jersey.

An outbreak of measles that was found to have originated from Disneyland was recently reported (January 2015). It is now spreading not only through Southern California but into neighboring states and Mexico as visitors exposed to the infected child/family are returning home from vacation and spreading measles into their communities.

According to the news report, approximately 50 people in four states have been diagnosed to date, and that is only from initial exposure within the middle to end of December! The incubation period for measles is approximately 7 to 21 days following exposure.

An ER physician in New York (Robert Glatter from Lenox Hill Hospital, is quoted as saying that the outbreak "has the potential to develop into one of the worse outbreaks since 1989."

Why? Because many parents are no longer vaccinating their children. Did you know that as of the year 2000, measles had been effectively eradicated from the United States? Now it's back. Around the world, according to World Health Organization, as stated in the article, thousands (approximately 75,000) from the Philippines and Vietnam had been infected and diagnosed. This may be the result of popular anti-vaccination attitudes not only in the US but around the world.

Misperceptions

We're not making an argument here of pro versus con. We're merely attempting to present both ends of the argument regarding vaccination against pertussis (or other preventable-disease vaccinations) so that you have the knowledge and the tools to continue your own research and make your own determination.

It's often difficult to know what to believe because when you look on the Internet or read certain books, depending on approach, you either have an extreme pro view or an extreme anti view presentation of facts, myths, information, as well as input from society at large.

There will be times when people will believe what they wish to believe regardless of scientific proof, facts, or studies, but that's a personal decision. However, in this section, we do want to provide a brief overview of some of the most common misperceptions and concerns regarding vaccines.

The Centers for Disease Control and Prevention provide a vast amount of information regarding research, safety, and use of, immunization schedules, and other facts that every parent needs to know about vaccines and immunizations. So too does the Mayo Clinic, the United States Public Health Department, the National Institutes of Health, and other agencies.

We urge every parent to take the time to sit down and research these documents, journal articles, and more for all the information you need, benefits as well as drawbacks, associated with any new drug, vaccine, or procedure.

Be an informed medical consumer, and do not make decisions based on common attitudes or opinions. Research the topics on your own and come to your own conclusion. Only then will you feel confident that you have made the right decision, whether you decide to immunize or not.

However, let's take a moment to discuss further a few of the most common misconceptions regarding vaccines mentioned by consumers today. First, we'll start off by saying that some of the most common mild reactions to a vaccine include soreness at the injection site, slight swelling, tenderness, and sometimes, a mild reaction evidenced by low-grade fevers. You should know that all of these reactions indicate that the vaccine is working.

However, you also need to be aware that your child may experience an allergic reaction, which occurs in approximately one out of every million children vaccinated. We briefly mentioned this earlier. However, we reiterate that no verifiable, statistical, or clinical evidence that links vaccinations to autism or any other neurological condition or disease process has been verified by clinical studies and/or data.

Remember that vaccinations can take a decade or more to develop, and governments around the world take extreme measures to ensure that the vaccinations have not only been proven to be effective, but are as safe as possible.

At the other end of the spectrum, you have the results and the effects that an infectious disease can have on children. Some of the risks of not vaccinating can include severe repercussions such as brain damage or even death. Be aware that the longer a parent delays vaccinating their children, the longer that child is exposed to risks of quite serious and often potentially life-altering diseases - even those that are preventable.

Another concern of parents is that a vaccine can literally overload a child's immune system. However, as briefly mentioned earlier, a baby's immune system, as that of children, are perfectly capable of receiving vaccinations according to the schedule recommended by government agencies as well as pediatricians around the world.

The American Academy of Pediatrics states that children, toddlers, and even babies' immune systems are more than capable of handling recommended vaccines based on standardized vaccination schedules.

That's because babies, no matter how careful you are to keep them isolated, are exposed to dozens if not hundreds of germs on a daily basis from the moment of birth.

According to the American Academy of Pediatrics, an infant's immune system is capable of responding to roughly 100,000 organisms at the same time.

You will note that the antigens found in vaccines only contain very small fractions of the response mechanisms required by a baby's immune system.

In fact, the immunization schedule is designed to protect children at their most susceptible young age after the natural immunity provided by their mother wears off following birth.

In addition, the American Academy of Pediatrics as well as the CDC aim to emphasize to parents that vaccinations do not weaken a body's immune system, or make a child sick with the disease they are being vaccinated against.

They are designed to deliver a disabled antigen of that disease into the body's immune system so that the immune system can naturally produce anti-bodies against it, creating immunity.

Let's focus again, briefly, on the myth that vaccinations cause autism. To date, there is no link to verify this statement, not only including autism, but other developmental disorders. A number of authoritative organizations in the United States and around the world have agreed that vaccinations are not only safe, but save lives. These include:

American Medical Association

American Academy of Family Physicians American Academy of Pediatrics

Centers for Disease Control and Prevention

Canadian National Advisory Committee on Immunization Department of Health of the United Kingdom

Gates Foundation

National Association for Pediatric Nurse Practitioners Infectious Diseases Society of America

European Center for Disease Prevention and Control Department of Health of the United Kingdom UNICEF

None of these groups have found any evidence to date, after reviewing more than 600 test cases and reports with no scientific or verifiable evidence that links vaccinations to autism.

Note: It should be noted by parents however, that autism does begin to present at the point in life when children do tend to receive their typical childhood vaccinations, and many parents mistakenly connect the two events. Access the footnote referring to Healthy Children Organization for some interesting reading regarding vaccines and neurological conditions like autism.

In fact, a great deal of this myth was perpetuated by a former doctor named Andrew Wakefield, who publicized his report by claiming a connection between vaccines and autism.

This doctor was later stripped of his license due to unethical behavior, and multiple sources determined that his study had been falsified.
However, the damage was done, and his report increased anxiety regarding the claimed link between autism and vaccination. As a result, this led to uninformed parents perpetuating the myth.

After Wakefield's article was published in the late 1990s, parents not only feared pertussis vaccinations, but also others, including measles and mumps.

To attempt a turnaround to this misnomer and alarming trend, the General Medical Council in England investigated these claims and in 2010 determined that Wakefield had engaged in deliberate fraud and based his research on bad science.

Hopefully, this information will serve to help parents make educated choices regarding vaccination.

Yes, babies are born with some immunity received from their mothers, but within a few months that immunity begins to wear off.

Babies are specifically protected from a variety of serious diseases, including pertussis, through vaccinations, because otherwise, they will not have any opportunity for their immune systems to build up any antibodies against such vaccine preventable diseases.

To reiterate, the earlier pertussis vaccine (DTP) that was first introduced in the 1940s was gradually phased out throughout the 1990s because of side effects that included fevers and some seizures.

It was at this time that the vaccine movements began, mainly because of the side effect of the endotoxin that was present in the membranes of the bacteria cells that created the vaccine.

It was at this time too that the DTaP vaccine was created, providing a number of benefits of the older vaccine, without the side effects. However, it has become clear over time, due to the rising incidents of pertussis, that this vaccine has not been as effective as the older one, although it does come with benefits of protection as well as reducing the symptoms and severity of the disease. It's also prevented many deaths, the potential spread of the disease, as well as reducing the risk of re-infection.

It might also be worth mentioning that, while many of us carefully read the ingredients in our food products, we don't tend to read package inserts when it comes to medications, and the same can be said of vaccination consent forms.

Today, parents no longer have to sign forms for vaccinations. Most of us can say, "We don't know what's in the vaccine/s so I don't want my child to have it." However, you CAN find out what's in these vaccines, and it's something that every parent should be doing. Don't allow yourself to be swayed in one direction or the other without finding out for yourself. This is responsible parenthood.

It pays to be informed, regardless of which side of the "argument" regarding vaccinations you happen to be on. Many vaccines contain similar ingredients, which can include but are not limited to:

Weakened or inactivated cells of the virus or bacteria. A variety of additives are often included in vaccine production and can include but are not limited to sterile water, fluids containing protein, and saline; all used as suspension fluids. A number of preservatives as well as components that help stabilize the vaccines may include but are not limited to albumin, phenols, and glycine. For example, aluminum or aluminum salts or gels are often added as an adjuvant to increase the efficiency and stimulation of the vaccine. These adjuvants, according to the CDC, initiate an increased potency and earlier response mechanism as well as a stronger and persistent immune response.

A number of chemicals known as adjuvant/s increase immune reactions. In some cases, this adjuvant can be aluminum sulfide, aluminum hydroxide, aluminum, or something similar.

Antibiotics are often added to some vaccinations in order to prevent growth of bacteria during both production and storage stage. The CDC specifies that no vaccines produced in the United States contain penicillin.
Trace - emphasizing trace - amounts of thimerosal. This ingredient can be found in some flu vaccines, as well as the HiB and DTaP vaccinations. These trace amounts may be utilized in the actual manufacturing process. They are present in extremely minute amounts, but parents should be aware that there can be traces of this in the vaccination. Let's take this a bit further by stating that this ingredient has very low levels of danger because it is composed of ethylmercury, and not methylmercury.

Formaldehyde - most of us are familiar with this term when it comes to embalming and funerals, but keep in mind that formaldehyde is an organic compound that is found in many common and vastly used substances including nail polish, household products, and building materials. In vaccines, formaldehyde is an important ingredient because it literally inactivates bacterial products that are used for toxoid-type vaccines in order to create immunity. Formaldehyde is often utilized during the production process to kill undesired bacteria that might possibly contaminate the vaccination during the production process. Most traces of formaldehyde are extracted from the vaccine before it's packaged.

Human diploid cells - Okay, so viruses have to be grown in a living tissue. Human tissues may be utilized for this purpose.

Proponents against vaccinations claim that some cell lines still used today "may" date back to the 1950s, and "may" have mutated, therefore introducing foreign or unfamiliar DNA and RNA into babies.

Proponents against vaccinations may also focus on the fact that a virus or bacteria can be cultured or grown in an animal cellular structure, such as chicken embryos or monkey kidney cells. Hundreds of modern medicines and drugs are developed in the same way.

Eggs (the MMR vaccine contains some presence of eggs, so anyone with an allergy to eggs is contraindicated from obtaining the MMR vaccine). The egg proteins are typically found in yellow fever and influenza vaccines, and are prepared utilizing chicken eggs. Most individuals who are able to eat egg-products or eggs without any allergic reactions are able to receive these two vaccinations.

Neomycin - a common and highly used antibacterial agent found in most vaccines.

Some immunizations contain MSG (monosodium glutamate, a known neurotoxin found in, for example, FluMist, a flu nasal spray). Monosodium glutamate is often utilized as a stabilizer in some vaccines to prevent any alteration to the vaccine due to humidity, exposure to light, heat, and acidity.

The CDC also states that numerous agencies including the Centers for Disease Control and Prevention, the Food and Drug Administration, the National Institutes of Health, as well as additional federal agencies, monitor and engage in research on a routine basis to carefully study and examine any newly broached evidence that even suggests the possibility of problems with the efficacy and/or safety of vaccines.

There are a number of sources including websites across the Internet that commonly propose that many ingredients in vaccines are extremely toxic. These sources are counted among the anti- vaccination camp, and do promote the sounding of the alarm bells, we are presenting both pros and cons, so we also have to take the time to present some of these more common statements.

For example, a website that classifies itself as a natural health news and self-reliance site states that toxic ingredients in vaccines as well as their adverse side effects include (based on the terminology of that website):

Sorbitol - a synthetic sweetener that is believed to be slowly metabolized by the body and can exacerbate irritable bowel syndrome as well as other gastrointestinal issues.

Bovine cow serum - this serum is extracted from cow skin and can cause chest pain, connective tissue disorders, arthritis, lupus, low blood pressure, skin reactions, and shortness of breath.

Sodium chloride - may increase blood pressure as well as restrict muscle growth and contraction capability.

Gelatin - collagen derivative from animal bone and skin. Increases the risk of infection due to synthetic growth hormones or even Mad Cow Disease.

Formaldehyde - fluid utilized to embalm corpses, and can cause liver damage, reproductive information, respiratory distress, cancer, and gastrointestinal issues. The website also states that formaldehyde is known to deactivate the virus that the vaccine has been created to cure, enabling live virus to enter the blood and infect the system (no resource for that statement was given).

Aluminum phosphate - huge potential for increasing mercury toxicity, with an emphasis on caution regarding minimum mercury tolerance that they believe that CDC scientists, as well as doctors are well aware of, and have seriously underestimated.

MSG - when utilized in injections, can become a neurotoxin, causing central nervous system disorders and even brain damage in children.

Never mind the fact that MSG is a common food preservative and ingredient found in a wide variety of food products and in restaurant usage today. The same goes for gelatin and sorbitol. Most people are not affected by monosodium glutamate, although some who are more susceptible may experience migraine headaches.

It should be noted that the levels of any of these ingredients are at such a minimal dosage that it would be quite rare to develop toxicity to any of them. For example, it is claimed that sorbitol leads to severe gastrointestinal problems, but the amount needed to cause that distress is measured at approximately 50 g+ for an adult. Increased levels of sorbitol in cellular structures can cause damage, and can aggravate conditions involving fructose malabsorption as well as irritable bowel syndrome.

Now when it comes to the sorbitol mentioned in the MMR vaccine, it's important to not only understand the ingredients, but the dosage. Four major vaccines given for the MMR vaccine (MMRII, Attenuvax, Mumpsvax, and MeruvaxII) all give dosages of the vaccine at approximately 0.5mL.

The amount of sorbitol contained in such dosages is measured at approximately 14.5 mg, well under the maximum required to initiate gastrointestinal distress as mentioned above.

The CDC publishes (last updated September 2013) ingredients included in vaccines produced in the United States. It is public knowledge that takes a little research to find.

These ingredients not only include benign vaccine ingredients such as preservatives and adjuvants, but any substances utilized during the manufacturing process. This includes any vaccine production media that are removed or extracted from the final product and are ultimately present in trace quantities. That said, it should be noted that most vaccines produced in the United States today do contain a low level of table salt (sodium chloride).

Let's take a closer look at the exact ingredients in several of the most common formulations of the pertussis vaccine:

DTaP (Daptacel) - aluminum phosphate, formaldehyde, glutaraldehyde, 2-Phenoxyethanol, Stainer-Scholte medium, modified Mueller's growth medium, modified Mueller-Miller casamino acid medium (without beef heart infusion), dimethyl 1-beta-cyclodextrin, ammonium sulfate.

DTaP (Infanrix) - formaldehyde, glutaraldehyde, aluminum hydroxide, polysorbate 80, Fenton medium (containing bovine extraction), modified Latham medium (derived from bovine casein) modified Stainer-Scholte liquid medium.

DTaP-IPV (Kinrix) – formaldehyde, glutaraldehyde, aluminum hydroxide, Vero (monkey kidney) cells, calf serum, lactalbumin hydrolysate, polysorbate 80, neomycin sulfate, polymixin B,

Fenton medium (containing bovine extract) modified Latham medium (derived from bovine casein), modified Stainer-Scholte liquid medium.

DTaP-HepB-IPV (Pediarix) - formaldehyde, glutaraldehyde, aluminum hydroxide, aluminum phosphate, lactalbumin hydrolysate, polysorbate 80, neomycin sulfate, polymyxin B, yeast protein, calf serum, Fenton medium (containing bovine extract), modified Latham medium (derived from bovine casein), modified Stainer-Scholte liquid medium, Vero (monkey kidney) cells.

DTaP-IPV/Hib (Pentacel) - aluminum phosphate, polysorbate 80, formaldehyde, glutaraldehyde, bovine serum albumin, 2-phenoxethanol, neomycin, polymyxin B sulfate, Mueller's Growth Medium, Mueller-Miller casamino acid medium (without beef heart infusion), Stainer-Scholte medium (modified by the addition of casamino acids and dimethyl-beta-cyclodextrin), MRC-5 (human diploid) cells, CMRL 1969 medium (supplemented with calf serum), ammonium sulfate, and medium 199.

Tdap (Adacel) - aluminum phosphate, formaldehyde, glutaraldehyde, 2-phenoxyethanol, ammonium sulfate, Stainer-Scholte medium, dimethyl-beta-cyclodextrin, modified Mueller's growth medium, Mueller-Miller casamino acid medium (without beef heart infusion).

Tdap (Boostrix) - formaldehyde, glutaraldehyde, aluminum hydroxide, polysorbate 80 (Tween 80), Latham medium derived from bovine casein, Fenton medium containing a bovine extract, Stainer-Scholte liquid medium.

As mentioned above, it's important not only to know of the

components of DTaP vaccines, but the dosage and concentration of excipients so that you can make an educated and rational decision regarding their safety and/or efficacy. Here's a breakdown of the basic dosage and milligrams of the most common components of the DTaP vaccines.

Dosage: 0.5mL Excipients:

Daptacel - formaldehyde, 0.1 mg glutaraldehyde, 50ng (nano grams) Adjuvant - aluminum phosphate, 0.33 mg Preservative per dose – 2-Phenoxyehtanol, 3.3 mg (0.6% v/v)

Infanrix –formaldehyde, 100 mcg polysorbate 80, 100 mcg sodium chloride, 4.5 mg per milliliter (4.5mg/mL) Adjuvant - aluminum hydroxide, 0.625 mg Preservative – none

Kinrix - formaldehyde, 100 mcg polysorbate 80, 100 mcg sodium chloride, 4.5 mg

Adjuvant - aluminum hydroxide, 0.6 mg Preservative - none Let's talk a minute about some of these ingredients and focus a moment on formaldehyde. Formaldehyde, as mentioned earlier, is most known as an embalming agent, but it's also found in wrinkle-free fabrics, cosmetics including hair styling products, nail polish removers, and nail polish. It's also found in furniture building materials including plywood, particle board, compressed wood, and many lacquered pieces of furniture.

Formaldehyde is a natural product produced in small amounts by our bodies and is part of our normal metabolism. Certain levels of formaldehyde are also found in not only the foods we consume, but in the air we breathe at work, as well as at home, and a number of products that we even rub into our skin.

Formaldehyde is also a byproduct of cigarettes and tobacco products, and is often used as a preservative in Italian cheeses, fish, and dried foods. It can be found in everything from dishwashing liquid to carpet cleaners, cosmetics, medicines, and fabric softeners.

Formaldehyde is quickly broken down by the body, and nearly every tissue in the human body is capable of breaking down the components of formaldehyde. It then converts it to a non-dangerous or non-toxic chemical in the body called formate, which is in turn excreted from the body in urine.

In addition, your lungs can convert formaldehyde into carbon dioxide. In some cases, your body may utilize formaldehyde to create larger molecules in the body that attach to DNA (deoxyribonucleic acid) as well as to certain proteins in the body.

Formaldehyde is not used in the production of any live virus vaccine such as MMR, rotavirus, some flu vaccines, and Varicella vaccines, or they would be rendered useless.

Only inactivated vaccines can utilize formaldehyde in the production process. Then, once the virus or bacteria is inactivated, the formaldehyde is diluted out of it, leaving only very trace or minute amounts.

So exactly how much formaldehyde is contained in pertussis vaccines? Measurements are defined in µg (microgram)/dose. Here's a breakdown:

Infantrix contains (100)

Daptacel contains (5)

Pediatrix and Kinrix each contain (100) Pentacel contains (5) Formaldehyde can be dangerous to life at a level of 20 ppm or parts per million, or at 0.2 mg per kilogram of body weight every day, with chronic exposure.

Proponents against the vaccination also claim that the ingredients listed above might cause rather severe allergic reactions, and the body might also store trace amounts of mercury and/or aluminum aflatoxin, which eventually, and if in high enough amounts, can lead to neurological conditions.

However, according to the CDC, the body is able to metabolize most heavy metals in a timely manner. Again, someone with a compromised immune system or deficient metabolism may not metabolize these metals as efficiently.

While some parents may focus on these ingredients in a negative way, we must also remember that many of the products and foods we eat today contain much higher levels of "dangerous" components, chemicals, and ingredients than those that are found in a common vaccination.
How is Safety of Vaccines Determined?

Let's take a closer look at how the safety of vaccines are monitored, case in point, by the Centers for Disease Control and Prevention (CDC.) For example, in the United States, the CDC continually monitors the safety of vaccines through a variety of systems. If and when any vaccine is determined to lead to health problems, the vaccine is studied and withdrawn from the public.

Due to improving technology and tracking, vaccines are now developed even for those who have higher risks of interactions or complications including the elderly, pregnant women, as well as those diagnosed with a chronic medical condition. So how does the CDC monitor vaccination safety?

We'll delve into deeper detail regarding the clinical trials that are undertaken before a vaccine is licensed. As mentioned earlier, vaccines are tested first on adults, utilizing anywhere between 20 and 100 healthy adult test subjects during the Phase I trials. They receive the vaccine, and then the researchers determine answers to certain questions, which include:

Does the vaccine appear to work?

Is it safe?

Are any serious side effects noted?

In relation to the side effects, does it have anything to do with the size of the dose?

During the Phase II trials, the test is then given to several hundred more volunteers, and the researchers will study the results and answer additional questions which may include:

What are the most common, short-term side effects that have been noted with the vaccine?

How did the immune systems of the volunteers respond to the vaccination?

During the Phase III clinical trials, hundreds, and sometimes even thousands of additional volunteers participate, with some of the questions providing focus for researchers that may include but are not limited to:

a) Identifying the data and comparing between those that

do get the vaccine and those that don't.

b) Does the vaccine still appear to be safe?

c) Does the vaccine still appear to be effective?

d) Again, the researchers will want to identify the most common side effects experienced by the test subjects

In the United States, the Federal Drug Administration (FDA) will only issue a license for a vaccine if it's considered effective, safe, and its benefits outweigh the risks. Every lot produced by manufacturers is tested for purity, potency, and safety. These lots will only be released for public dissemination after the FDA has previewed their quality standards as well as safety.

We encourage parents to visit the website of the FDA at www.fda.gov/cber for more information on how they inspect the manufacturing process, as well as the facilities, in order to maintain their standard of quality and safety.

After the Food and Drug Administration has licensed a vaccine, then medical experts and health authorities will consider adding the vaccine to a recommended schedule of immunizations. This is done by the Advisory Council on Immunization Practices (in the US), made up of a cluster of the public as well as medical health experts.

In addition, other members of the health profession, including those of the American Academy of Family Physicians and the American Academy of Pediatrics, will also be among some of the groups that will bring their knowledge, expertise, and input to that committee.

The group will then thoroughly review all the available data that has been compiled regarding the vaccine studies as well as clinical trials before they make recommendations for the vaccine. How do they make these recommendations? They assess a variety of factors, including:

a) Determining the safety of the vaccine at specific age groups.

b) Determining the efficacy of the vaccine in specific age groups.

c) Assessing the seriousness of the disease that the vaccine is designed to prevent.

d) Determining how many children would be at risk for contracting the disease that the vaccine is designed to prevent, if the vaccine were not made available.

Even after these assessments, the recommendations of the Advisory Council on Immunization Practices is not considered completed or official until the Director of the CDC reviews and proves these results and they are published.

Only after this process will recommendations regarding vaccines or their inclusion in immunization schedules become a part (in the United States) of the official and recommended childhood immunization schedule.

Even after the vaccine has been added to the recommended immunization schedule, experts in a variety of health fields will continue to oversee and monitor the effectiveness as well as the safety of the vaccine.

This same process is followed by different organizations and structures, throughout the world.

Monitoring Safety

How does the CDC, the FDA, or other global organizations monitor the safety and effectiveness of vaccines after they've been disseminated to the public? In fact, why do they need to be monitored anyway if they've gone through such rigorous testing standards?

The reason that governmental agencies and health experts continue to monitor vaccines is to note any possible side effects, as well as ensuring that any risks linked to the vaccine are quickly identified. One of the major organizations responsible for this in the United States is the Vaccine Adverse Event Reporting System or VAERS. This organization assimilates, collects, and analyzes data and reports of adverse effects that occur following vaccination. Healthcare professionals, patients themselves, and parents can submit their reports to this organization.

In addition to VAERS, a network of professional health care organizations throughout the United States (the Vaccine Safety Datalink or VSD) is also available to the public for a variety of healthcare information.

This organization is a valuable resource for scientists and medical researchers in engaging studies that continually evaluate the efficacy as well as safety of vaccines. If safety monitoring and oversight shows that any vaccine does carry risks that outweigh benefits, the recommendations for the vaccine may be changed.

In addition to the two organizations mentioned above, a third, the Clinical Immunization Safety Assessment network (CISA), also monitors safety activities. In a nutshell:

The Vaccine Adverse Effect Reporting System (VAERS) is designed as an "early warning" system utilized by public health departments and is accessible by individuals who can report their concerns regarding vaccines. This organization helps the Federal Drug Administration and the Centers for Disease Control and Prevention in detecting possible side effects following a vaccination.

The Vaccine Safety Datalink (VSD) is an organization that collaborates with a variety of healthcare organizations as well as the Centers for Disease Control and Prevention to monitor as well as evaluate and analyze any side effects following vaccination that are reported.

The Clinical Immunization Safety Assessment network (CISA) is an organization that also collaborates between a variety of medical research centers in the United States as well as the Centers for Disease Control and Prevention to conduct further research into how many side effects or adverse events might be initiated by a vaccine.

Indeed, a variety of new and recent global immunization initiatives and vaccine safety monitoring processes continue to grow not only in the United States, but around the world.

Organizations such as those listed above are vitally important in the monitoring of vaccine safety.

Parents in the United States may feel comforted by the fact that the country has one of the safest vaccine supplies in history.

As a parent, it's important to know what's contained in the vaccines you give your children. This information is readily available from the Centers for Disease Control at their website at www.cdc.gov. It's important to rely on accurate and reliable data when it comes to such questions and issues. Your local Department of Public Health, the CDC, and other global organizations sponsored by the government are excellent resources for parents looking for information regarding the safety, efficacy, and durability of any kind of vaccination.

We'll talk more about natural approaches to treating whooping cough, some of which may be very effective, but it is also important to offer reliable and effective research for both sides of the argument. Yes, parents can buy organic minerals, vitamins, antioxidants, amino acids, and enzymes to promote overall health and wellness, but it's also important to acknowledge the efficacy of modern medicine when it comes to preventable disease vaccination and immunization schedules.

Why take a chance? When coupled together, combining alternative or natural approaches to disease prevention with vaccinations may provide optimal benefits for children, teenagers, and adults.

Take a look at some of just a few of the pro and con posts regarding vaccination for pertussis accessed during our research. Following are a few comments found on a variety of discussion boards regarding whooping cough vaccines and their safety:

"When I was younger and they tried to give me the whooping cough vaccine I got really sick and went into convulsions. It almost killed me, then when I got older my mom asked if I might have grown out of it and if they could try it again. But they said it was too risky. From what I've read, the old whooping cough vaccine used to cause seizures after a couple hours to some kids. So maybe I wasn't allergic to the vaccine. But I'm not sure, 'cause I don't know too much about the vaccine, because I could never have it and I was too young to remember. I am really tired of getting whooping cough almost every winter."

Here's another one: "My baby, at the age of eight weeks, had a toxic reaction to his central nervous system after an injection of the whooping cough vaccine. He cried and screamed off and on for 72 hours. He has never had another injection of the vaccine. He is 24 years old now and refuses the vaccine. He has never had whooping cough. But the thought of him trying it again concerns him and me greatly."

And another: "We have a new grandchild due at the end of the month. My daughter-in-law is insisting that all family members planning to have contact with the child must be current with their whooping cough vaccine. I see information on the web concerning the Tdap vaccine for adults 18 to 64, but nothing for us old folks. I am 69!"

In reply to the above post, the facilitator of the forum board replied, "Incidents of whooping cough are on the rise. It is pretty standard practice to require family members who might be around a newborn to get the vaccination. They are in the most at risk group if they are infected. I'm more familiar with the younger population and immunizations, other than those I need. I'd say it would be good to call and talk to your doctor or a local clinic. If that isn't a good option, maybe your daughter-in-law's doctor could advise you on whether or not it would be a good choice for you - you might also want to call your local health department. Even with the Internet, there are still a lot of voids out there."

Writes a forum board poster from California in 2010, "I thought I'd pass this along here. California has experienced an outbreak of pertussis (whooping cough) with 1,500 cases. Adults almost always recover, but it can be deadly for infants. Babies are not immune until after their final shot at six months. Therefore, it's imperative for all caregivers of infants to have a booster shot. Although this outbreak is in California, I get the booster no matter where I live."

And another poster: "Despite all the hype that illegal immigration is causing the outbreak in California, it has more to do with parents NOT immunizing their kids. It's unbelievable to me that parents can send their kids to school without vaccinations, endangering the health of everyone else."

Another parent writes, "I just don't get the parents who don't vaccinate their children. I mean I understand that there is so many different things and no shots, but if it's going to protect my child against something that could be so harmful to him, it just makes sense."

And another: "It's not only kids who aren't vaccinated, but they are also finding out that the shots many of us received as children may not be protecting us enough and we therefore can be carriers of pertussis. I have made all my family members get the adult vaccination. It includes the pertussis booster and tetanus shot in one."

As you can see, the opinions and stance on vaccination, both pros and cons, is prevalent in society today, and is likely to stay. However, that being said, we urge parents to dig into the research. Be wary of what you read if statistics or comments aren't backed up by resources or verified.

You can go online and look at articles and even books written by apparently credible authors, but parents reading a book/article/brochure should not just believe everything at face value.

For example, one book on vaccines that strove to provide parents with enough information to make an informed decision regarding vaccines for their children, received negative customer reviews (we will not name it due to ethical reasons). Several of these reviews pointed out a variety of negative aspects, listing items like studies that were cited didn't support the claims in the book, to one-sided points of view as well as bad science.

One of the reviews stated that the book cited a study from the New England Journal of Medicine, a certainly reputable medical journal in the industry. The author of the book (we're not here to discredit any authors, but are emphasizing reliability and accuracy) claimed that he had referenced an article stating that there was a link found between polio vaccines and paralysis.

However, when the reviewer actually looked up the resource and read the actual text of the referenced study, they discovered that the study did not imply this. The reviewer then made a very good suggestion in that anyone reading a heavily cited book referenced through footnotes or case studies should actually read them.

Another person, a scientist, had these comments to make about this one particular book. "My wife just got this book and although I don't usually write reviews, I will make an exception on this one. I am a scientist and I am appalled at how bad the science in this book is. It is filled with fallacies, made-up facts, et cetera. Here is a short list:

Amish don't get vaccinated and they don't get autism: wrong. This is a well debunked myth. Amish do vaccinate, albeit to a lesser extent than the main population and they also get autism, independent of whether they were vaccinated or not.

Death from vaccines were decreasing before the development of vaccines. Although this is true (medical care was improving), what it does not say is that the incidence of diseases such as measles, polio, etc. significantly dropped after the introduction of vaccines. Medical care has improved such that people can survive polio, but please look at images of children who had polio and decide for yourself if you want your child to be like that.

VAERS is a database where anybody can report any event they think may be caused by vaccines. The analysis of reports versus what is expected by pure chance alone shows that most of these reports are not caused by vaccines. No researcher uses VAERS to derive any kind of conclusion, except the authors of this book apparently.

It cites Andrew Wakefield. This one is a kicker. If you ask my research fellows to name the worst scientist, Andrew Wakefield has to be at the top of that list. All his research has been discredited. Not only was he a bad researcher, we now know he was also a crook and a fraud."

About the same book, another reviewer wrote, "Two of the doctors whose research is cited in this book have been stripped of their licenses to practice medicine. (Mr. Wakefield for breach of professional ethics). The evidence of him falsifying research data was found later."

The point we're trying to make here is to do your best to obtain unbiased and "both sides of the fence" information, data, and research that helps you come to your own decision of whether to vaccinate or not. It is a personal decision, and both sides of the argument deserve respect and attention.

Chapter Five: Treating Whooping Cough

Now that we've discussed what whooping cough is, how the condition progresses, and the pros and cons of vaccinations, let's get down to the nitty-gritty - treating whooping cough.

Today, treating whooping cough can take two different approaches, and we're not talking about vaccinating or not vaccinating here. We're talking about how to care for a child, a teen, or an adult who contracts whooping cough. What are your options for treatment?

The mainstay of treatment is providing supportive care. Some approaches today use antibiotics, or natural or "alternative" approaches. Whether you decide to go holistic or homeopathic, know and understand your options.

Let's first explore the traditional or conventional approach to treatment of whooping cough, which may involve the use of antibiotics. We'll break this down based on the age of the patient: infant, toddler, child, teenager, and adult.

Traditional treatment for whooping cough is generally supportive, and in some cases, may involve the use of antibiotics. If you get treatment early enough, you may experience less severe symptoms, and sometimes avoid getting coughing fits.

However, beyond the first three weeks of developing symptoms, antibiotics are not as useful, and it's likely that you'll just have to let the condition run its course.

Several anti-microbial treatments are recommended by the CDC, but early identification and treatment is highly recommended. Even when it comes to infants, the earlier the diagnosis, and the earlier initiation of treatment, the better. For example, the CDC states that if treatment is started within the first week or two of initiation of coughing episodes or paroxysms, the symptoms can be reduced.

As mentioned in an earlier chapter, an individual with whooping cough is considered infectious from the beginning of the catarrhal stage, or the point in time where you notice a runny nose, the low- grade fever, and the sneezing (basically, the symptoms of a common cold). Infectiousness continues up to about the third week, and after the onset of coughing fits or the multiple, rapid coughs known as paroxysms. The patient will also stop being contagious approximately five days after the beginning of an effective anti-microbial treatment.

The CDC emphasizes and supports targeted post-exposure antibiotics and anti-microbial prophylaxis for use in individuals who are at high risk of developing severe pertussis, and have come into close contact with persons affected by pertussis.

The three major anti-microbial agents in the treatment of pertussis include:

1) Erythromycin

2) Azithromycin

3) Clarithromycin

Trimethoprim-sulfamethoxasole may also be used.

The decision of which antimicrobial to use is often determined by the pediatrician or doctor based on:

a)   The ability of the infant/child/person to tolerate a particular antimicrobial

b)   Possibility for certain 'adverse' affects as well as drug interactions (if the individual is already taking another drug/medication)

c)   Cost

d)   Ability of parent or caregiver to follow the recommended or prescribed regimen or plan of care

According to the CDC, erythromycin, clarithromycin, and azithromycin are recommended (and preferred) for the treatment of pertussis in those over the age of one month. For those under this age, azithromycin is most recommended for post-exposure treatment and prophylaxis.

Parents can learn more about antimicrobials by accessing the CDC website at: http://www.cdc.gov/pertussis/clinical/treatment.html

Note: Azithromycin may be contraindicated for some elderly or patients with cardiac issues. If you or a loved one fits such a category, talk to your doctor or healthcare provider prior to receiving the antimicrobial.

Parents today should know that earlier, phased out vaccines contained whole cell bacterial (dead) along with detoxified components of diphtheria and tetanus particles, literally containing many components designed to stimulate immune system function.

The more current vaccines (acellular versions) contain fragments of pertussis although with the endotoxin removed. As such, they provide only one to four antigens that stimulate the immune system rather than the dozens that were utilized in the old vaccine.

Interestingly, studies have shown that the endotoxin originally used in the old vaccines provided the greatest benefit and more powerful and long-lasting immune responses, even though it did come with more side effects. As such, modern society is met with a conundrum. At what point do we go so far as to create vaccines with the fewest side effects while producing those very same vaccines without the efficacy they offered in older vaccines? This is a matter best left to the researchers and scientists, but is something that every parent should consider as well.

About Natural Remedies and Approaches to Care

A number of natural and herbal remedies are recommended by parents who have tried the alternative approach to care for whooping cough. However, it is suggested that whether you decide to vaccinate or not, that if your child contracts whooping cough, do discuss your use of herbal or natural remedies with the pediatrician involved in your child's care, especially if your child is taking antibiotics. This is because a number of herbal remedies found not only in nature, but also in synthetic remedies, as well as in natural food supply and health stores, may interact with antibiotics, and either reduce efficacy, or can create unintended complications.

One of the greatest concerns of parents taking care of a child with whooping cough is the cough itself. It's hard, spasmodic, and painful. Additionally, a huge amount of mucus secretions may be produced through coughing, and you may literally see this mucus running from the nose. However, if you decide to go the natural route, you'll find a number of herbal remedies or holistic treatments that can not only speed recovery, but help to ease the cough.

Such treatments and remedies may help with other common childhood illnesses including coughs, and pain and fever associated with flu bugs and other illnesses.

Again, always let your pediatrician know that you are trying such treatments, and be able to specify the ingredients as well as amounts of those ingredients that you are offering to your child. This also includes information about dosages, as well as how many times a day you are giving (or intending to give) your child the natural remedy or treatment based on label instructions. Better yet, take the remedy to your doctor so they can see exactly what it is and explain dosing recommendations based on weight and age.

One of the most common herbs used to treat coughs was also used by the Plains Indians of the Americas. They commonly sought out marshmallow root, which they either dried or used fresh, mixing with a variety of liquids and taken as a tea-like substance. This treatment is not medically supported, and is not based on verifiable evidence for efficacy. (Keep in mind however, that
your pediatrician may recommend that you do not provide milk if your child is on antibiotics – as it can reduce the efficacy of some.)

Another proposed (and not medically supported and without verifiable evidence) natural remedy states that you can also use boiled water when making a tea out of marshmallow root. This root works by encouraging the body to create a thin film of mucus that coats the throat as well as the bronchial tubes, relieving the sensation of itching or "tickling" that can trigger a coughing spasm. Not only that, but marshmallow root can soothe irritated membranes and reduce the frequency and intensity of coughing.

Another common herb often used as an expectorant is Lobelia inflata. This herb is often used as a natural and beneficial expectorant that will help to relieve the chronic and deep cough produced by the whooping cough bacteria. It is also believed to be effective at loosening up mucus that can help to relieve congestion in the airways and the chest.

Note: This herb is often used in a combination form of herbal cough tonics. Never use it on its own, as it is toxic! That means that parents should not go into a health food store and utilize this herb in any form of self-treatment. Instead, consult a practitioner who is educated and knowledgeable regarding herbal medicine, so do follow appropriate guidelines for its use.

Steaming. We have all seen the images on TV or in magazines of people leaning over bowls, kettles, or parts of steaming water with a towel over their head. This is a form of holistic medicine that has been used for generations, and even thousands of years, to relieve coughing and to loosen phlegm and mucus. When combined with herbal remedies, steaming can stimulate not only the immune system, but loosen up stubborn coughs.

You don't have to place or hold your child over a pot full of steaming water. You can create the same effect in your bathroom. For example, take the child into the bathroom, close the doors and turn on the shower, using only hot water.

Allow the steam produced by the hot water to fill the bathroom. Of course, if you'd rather not waste the water, fill a bowl, pot, or other container with hot water and then place a towel over the bowl as well as your child's head to create a makeshift "steam tent." For added benefit, you may even wish to place a few drops of lavender oil into the water, or eucalyptus oil to help break up the cough and provide a soothing aroma.

Note: Use caution any time you have your child or an infant around hot water. Make sure that the steam is not hot enough to burn their tender skin. Like testing milk for temperature, place the inside of your wrist over the bowl when covered with a towel to make sure it's not too hot.

Parents should also be cautioned not to use eucalyptus oil if the child is also taking or using other homeopathic remedies, as it can make them ineffective. Again, if you decide to try a steam treatment, let your pediatrician know ahead of time.

When it comes to homeopathic remedies, approach with knowledge and caution. Though the evidence perspective is lacking, many believe that homeopathy can provide a number of benefits for a wide variety of illnesses, but you have to know what you are doing.

Homeopathy is classified as an alternative form of medicine. It typically believes that "like treats like" - it's a practice and philosophy that is literally based on the idea that the body, with the help of natural herbal formulas, tinctures, and remedies, can heal itself.

In its "modern form" homeopathy has been practiced since the late 1700s, originating in Germany. Basically, homeopathy takes the view that the illness or symptoms of illnesses are typical and very normal responses of the human body that is attempting to heal itself.

A homeopath, or homeopathic health practitioner, can utilize a variety of solutions (liquid mixtures), pills, or other formulas that contain extremely small amounts of active ingredients typically found in mineral or plant form in the treatment of diseases. These formulas, which are extremely diluted, are known as potentiated substances.

You may be relieved to know that since the late 1930s, numerous homeopathic remedies have been regulated and overseen by numerous agencies in the US, and are considered to be generally safe.

However, because of the very small amount of active ingredients found in the remedies, some opponents of homeopathy believe that it creates nothing more than a placebo effect. Regardless, if you decide you want to try a homeopathic dilution or remedy on your child to help deal with the symptoms of whooping cough, do discuss your intentions with your doctor, because the preparations used by homeopathic practitioners may vary in strength as well as quality.

Again, any alternative treatment (and that goes for over-the- counter medicines too) can interact with traditional and conservative approaches to care, including the medications your child may be taking.

You should follow the recommendations of your doctor or pediatrician to avoid increased risks or concerns – this is your child, after all. In some cases, you may need to decide whether to rely on conventional or alternative therapies, and not combine the two.

Homeopathic Remedies

While we want to include this information, parents should be aware that these remedies are used by homeopaths, and as such as are not backed by verifiable evidence regarding their efficacy or safety.

One of the most common homeopathic remedies that a parent can use to deal with the spasmodic coughing fits experienced by those dealing with whooping cough is grindelia robusta, otherwise known as Rosin Wood or Gum Plant. This remedy didn't come into common practice in the United States until the mid-1800s after it became relatively known as a beneficial medicinal and therapeutic herb. The herb was listed in the Pharmacopeia of United States between 1882 and 1926.

As herbal infusion, this remedy is typically prepared by steeping roughly 1 teaspoonful of the dried herb into 1 cup of boiling water. However, when mixing this remedy, you must allow the tea to steep for approximately 10 to 15 minutes before sipping. It is often recommended twice daily.

Grindelia robusta is often used as a homeopathic remedy for not only dealing with conditions that create a dense mucus, but chronic bronchitis as well as asthma. It is known as a quite effective remedy for the wheezing caused by whooping cough, and by bronchitis. The tincture is often recommended in a dosage of 1 to 15 drops, but is also available in lower potencies. Again, don't guess! Talk to someone who is knowledgeable and experienced in homeopathy before grabbing such products off the shelf and just guessing at dosages.

Another common homeopathic remedy is drosera rotundifolia. This homeopathic remedy is designed to focus on the respiratory organs and has long been used as the most common remedy for whooping cough.

Also known as Sun Dew or Red Rot, the remedy is created by using a fresh and entire Sandhu plant in bloom. This remedy has been passed down from generation to generation of homeopathic healers and practitioners since the 16th century. The plant is typically chopped into very small pieces and then pounded into alcohol and then the solution is strained.

Note: It is not recommended by medical experts to use alcohol as a remedy in sick children with a potentially devastating illness/es.

Another common homeopathic remedy used to treat the dry, hard cough produced when phlegm is coughed out of the throat is bryonia. This herb, also known as White Bryony or Wild Hops, was used in ancient Greece and made its way toward Western Europe by the 1600s.

However, this remedy is only utilized in therapeutic environments because the plant itself can be extremely toxic. This remedy is used by preparing the root of the plant, and then beneficial "juices" are extracted by compressing root pulp with alcohol in the preparation of a very highly diluted solution.

Again, rely on educated and experienced homeopathic healers or doctors who do often combine more traditional treatments for illnesses with alternative forms of medicine including homeopathic remedies. Many of these formulas, tinctures, and products can be toxic if not used properly and should only be used in extremely small doses.

Taking Care of a Child with Whooping Cough

No doubt about it, chances are that your child is not the only one that's going to grow a little cranky when sick with whooping cough. Because coughing can last between two and three minutes (and last for weeks!), it can be quite distressing not only for the child, but for a parent having to watch the child endure these coughing fits. In many cases, you may notice that your child's face grows extremely red. Your child may vomit after the coughing fit.

How exactly do you provide comfort to a young child overcome with these coughing fits? How do you deal with them when they become cranky because they're exhausted not only from the coughing, but because they (and you) constantly wake up through the night because of the coughing?

Your child may lose weight because of a lack of appetite or because the coughing paroxysms cause vomiting, leading to inadequate nutrient intake. It may be difficult to feed a baby or toddler because of these coughing fits. So what's a parent to do?

As mentioned previously, bacteria cause whooping coughs, but once the coughing has started, antibiotics are not very effective in stopping the cough. Many parents look to cough suppressants to deal with this, but it's important to avoid their use. The child (or adult) needs to cough up the mucus in order to prevent pneumonia.

In most cases, a child's own immune system (especially if they have been vaccinated) will kick in to help fight the bacteria within three to four weeks, but it may take longer for the bronchioles (small breathing airway tubes) found in the lungs to heal.

When taking care of a child diagnosed with whooping cough, it's important to keep the child isolated from others, especially other children, for approximately three weeks. This is extremely beneficial in halting the spread of the infection. If your child has been given antibiotics (most commonly erythromycin), before the coughing fits have started, this seclusion can be limited to about a week. Always talk to your doctor about this.

Note: In events where antibiotics have been prescribed, it's important to give your child all the doses recommended by your doctor, even when you see improvement.

In the event that your child complains, or you see signs that the coughing is painful, you can give them paracetamol or ibuprofen to increase their comfort levels. Again, always follow the dosage instructions found on the packaging, as it can be dangerous to give infants, toddlers, or small children more than recommended amounts.

Encourage your child to rest as often as possible, and to eat a healthy, nutritious meal. In most cases, parents may find it more effective to feed young children right after the conclusion of a coughing spell to help keep drinks and food down. It has been noted that feeding a child who has not recently had a coughing fit can trigger a coughing spell.

Also keep in mind that your child may complain of stomach pain, which is understandable, given the fact that coughing can cause not only chest pain, but abdominal pain from the constant coughing.

Following are a few additional suggestions regarding care in home-based scenarios when it comes to treating whooping cough:

a) Do your best to keep the child hydrated, encouraging small sips of liquid on an hourly basis when they are awake. This will prevent dehydration. Offer whatever is tolerated, including water, fruit juice, or for older children, a decaffeinated sports drink which will help replace electrolytes lost through vomiting. Do not offer drinks that contain caffeine.

b) Eat small meals, and if you have to, encourage very small amounts of food, even when the child is not hungry. This will help to increase and maintain energy and strength.

c) Encourage rest. If your child is restless, try lying down with him or her to provide comfort and a sense of security.

d) Use a humidifier which may help to loosen the mucus in the upper chest and throat. Fill humidifiers with cool water. Talk to your pediatrician about safety use of humidifiers for infants, toddlers, or children diagnosed with pertussis.

e) If you live in the house of a smoker, discourage smoking, at least in the house while the child is sick (in any case, smoking should not occur inside the house at any time with children living there). You may also want to avoid use of wood burning fireplaces as exposure to smoke may increase the severity of coughing as well as increase difficulty in breathing.

What Caregivers have to Say

Following are a few comments, suggestions, and concerns of parents not only regarding exposure to whooping cough, but in providing care. The first one is from a young mother in Northern California:

"Coughing fits in babies are frightening to witness and may be triggered by mild stimulation such as startling sounds, feeding, or touching. Babies will become violently wracked by coughing fits and often take on a bluish-purple color due to a lack of oxygen.

Their eyes may bulge and water, cheeks may become flushed, they may stick out their tongue, push their chest forward and flail their limbs in distress. Many times infants will become markedly exhausted from the physical exertion of the coughing fits. The most serious risk is posed to infants four months of age and younger."

Writes an adult diagnosed with whooping cough: "The first couple of months are the worst, then it will gradually start getting better. I would cough so hard that I got lightheaded, vomited at times, pulled stomach muscles, hurt a rib, and had some incontinence. It was extremely hard to catch a breath in between the coughs. I was often bent over almost double while coughing. Things were worse for me because it was winter and I had cold air triggering my asthma cough too… I did keep sucking on mints, candy, cough drops, etc. to keep my mouth hydrated. I also made sure to drink tons of water to help. You will get through this, but it is miserable in the meantime. There really isn't anything else you can do other than endure."

Another adult rights, "I live in a college town. Two years ago whooping cough went through here like wildfire because by the time you get to college age, your immunity has worn off from the vaccination you received as a child. A friend of mine got it from his college-aged child, and he suffered for months, was put on steroids, but it just had to run its course. As far as the antibiotics causing stomach upset, if you will take acidophilus, you won't have the stomach upset. Just don't take the acidophilus at the same time you take the antibiotic. Take at least two hours after taking the antibiotic."

Providing Relief

So exactly how do you go about soothing a cranky child dealing with whooping cough? Caring for your toddler or small child when they're dealing with whooping cough is pretty much the same as you would for any illness that produces a cough. A few general standards apply, but again, discuss with your pediatrician. Here are a few basics:

Offer as many fluids as you can get your child to drink. This includes juice or water. Decaffeinated, warm tea may also help ease the tickling or the irritation that produces a cough. Warm liquids can also relieve coughing spasms. If your child is not allergic, add a teaspoon of honey to not only sweeten the tea, but to provide a soothing coating for an irritated throat.

If your child doesn't want to drink fluids, try sugar-free Popsicles. The cool Popsicle will not only provide some hydration, but will serve to soothe a reddened and irritated throat. As mentioned earlier, consider a humidifier, which adds moisture to the air.

Humidifiers are often effective, especially when you add eucalyptus or Vicks-type ointments to the water, which can help to loosen up congestion and mucus.

Again, if your child is not allergic to honey, offer a spoonful of honey before they go to bed. Honey is a wonderful substance that provides a coating and can help soothe the throat.

Note: Only give honey to children older than one year of age. In younger children and toddlers, honey can cause botulism.

Avoid the use of common cough medicines. Your first instinct may be to reach for the cough medicine, but the American Academy of Pediatrics as well as the US Food and Drug Administration urge parents to avoid their use for toddlers and infants. Not only are they not effective, but they can create a number of side effects, depending on the brand and dosage.

Also keep in mind that cough medicines that serve to suppress coughing may inhibit the ability of your child to fight off the infection. They can also cause drowsiness. In addition, cough medicines are rarely effective in reducing the frequency or severity of coughing, and those that contain dextromethorphan can actually produce a dry cough, which is not productive in removing the built-up mucus and congestion.

If your pediatrician does recommend a cough medication, it will most likely contain guaifenesin, such as Robitussin, which may make it easier for your child to cough up phlegm.

Note: When it comes to cough medications, follow precautions. Talk to your pediatrician before offering any cough medicine to children younger than six years of age.

We already mentioned steam tents, or taking your toddler or child into the bathroom where they can benefit from the steam produced by a hot shower. At the other end of the spectrum, you could try cool moist air, such as that found in the freezer. Try holding your child up to the freezer and opening the door, and having them inhale that cool air for a few minutes to see if it will help. In wintertime and in colder climates, you might also try taking your child outdoors, of course after bundling them up. The cool air often serves to soothe an irritated throat.

In any case where your child may look like they are struggling to breathe, or are coughing so hard that their lips turn blue, call your pediatrician or take your child to the emergency room as soon as possible. Bluish tinted skin around the mouth is a sign of lack of oxygen.

Ask your doctor, and if your toddler is old enough, whether you can give them acetaminophen and/or ibuprofen for relief of pain, discomfort, or low-grade fevers. Always remember that if your child has been prescribed antibiotics, give them to your child as directed.

Do not skip doses and do not stop providing the medication because the child may be feeling better. If the child seems to be growing worse, talk to your pediatrician before stopping the antibiotic.

You should also take some steps to reduce irritants in the home environment. Removing airborne irritants including pollen, molds, dust, and chemical fumes is essential. Keeping your air filters (and that includes air-conditioning and furnace filters) clean and changing them on a regular basis, can help cut down on airborne irritants in a home. Again, do your best to make sure that your child does not get exposed to secondary smoke.

It may also help to place another pillow under your child's shoulders and head while sleeping, and to encourage them to sleep on their left side, which can also help to reduce sensations of nausea. When it comes to reducing fever that often accompanies whooping cough, as mentioned, stick to:

Acetaminophen Ibuprofen (Advil, Motrin)
Naproxen (Aleve, Naprosyn, Anaprox)

Acetaminophen can help to decrease pain as well as fever, but will not help with any inflammation. The recommended dosage for acetaminophen is approximately 10 to 15 mg per kilogram of body weight (or 5 to 7 mg per pound) every four to six hours.

Parents are strongly urged not to exceed maximum daily dosage based on the age of the child. Also keep in mind that all acetaminophen products can come in a variety of strengths. Some of the most common acetaminophen products on the market today include Panadol and Tylenol.

Ibuprofen is effective in reducing fever, inflammation, and pain. It is classified as a non-steroidal anti-inflammatory medication also known as an NSAID. Recommended dosage for children over six months of age is approximately 7 to 10 mg per kilogram (4 to 5 mg per pound) of body weight, given every six hours. Some of the most popular brand names of ibuprofen include Motrin, Advil, and Nuprin.

Naproxen is effective in reducing inflammation, pain, and fever, and like ibuprofen is also a non-steroidal anti-inflammatory medication. This should only be given to children or teenagers or older persons in an approximate dosage of 200 mg twice a day, with food. Parents are cautioned not to exceed 500 mg of naproxen a day. The most popular brand name for naproxen is Aleve.

Again, watch for warning signs of whooping cough causing problems other than the general discomfort in your child. Some of the warning signs that you need to get your child to the doctor or to emergency services include:

a)   shortness of breath

b)   worsening of the cough

c) repetitive vomiting following a coughing spasm

d) cyanosis (blue lips or fingertips or the nail beds)

e) lethargy (excessive sleepiness)

f) confusion

Conclusion

The decision on whether to vaccinate your child or not, as well as how to provide care for a child or loved one who has contracted whooping cough, is not always a simple or a black-and-white issue.

Parents need to know about whooping cough and its possible effects on their child. At the same time, it's important for parents to educate themselves regarding vaccines and their use.

The argument regarding vaccinating or not vaccinating is likely to continue, depending on attitudes, geographical location, and even availability of vaccines. However, carefully weigh the pros and cons of making such a decision.

To reiterate, there are a number of points that parents or loved ones of someone who is at risk of contracting whooping cough should remember:

a) The cough associated with whooping cough can last as long as six months, sometimes even longer depending on the age, vaccination status and the overall general health and wellness of the child or teen or adult.

b) In severe cases of coughing spasms, which can often last

up to three minutes, your child may not only get very red in the face, but vomit after the coughing episode. It is very important to note that aspiration or inhaling vomit can cause severe issues in lung function, and can lead to pneumonia. In addition, a young infant who experiences such severe coughing spasms can literally be deprived of oxygen and go blue in the face due to a lack of oxygen.

c)   Whooping cough is serious, especially for infants, young children, and the elderly. It has caused death.

d)   Immunization greatly reduces the risk of children contracting whooping cough, and if they do, the durations and severity of the illness is less severe.

e)   When caring for children at home, keep them away from others, especially other children in the family or neighborhood for approximately three weeks. This will prove relatively effective in halting the spread of the infection.

Be aware of the more severe complications of whooping cough in babies and young children. These severe complications include:

a)   Lack of oxygen. Some infants and small children can stop breathing. Lack of oxygen can cause severe repercussions on the brain and other body functions. The longer the brain goes without oxygen, the more severe the repercussions.

b)   Pneumonia

c)   Seizures

d)   Bleeding into the brain, which can lead to brain damage.

In very young infants, whooping cough often presents with an unpredictable course, and some infants can rapidly decline or deteriorate. Following are a few alarming facts provided by kidshealth.org:

a) A baby under one year of age who is hospitalized with whooping cough has a 1 in 10 chance of requiring pediatric intensive care.

b) Infants placed in pediatric intensive care have a 1 in 6 chance of dying, or suffering lung damage or brain damage.

None of the information provided in this book is meant to sway parents one way or the other regarding getting or avoiding vaccines. It is important to know both the benefits and drawbacks of immunization, as well as what can happen if your child is not immunized.

Learn as much as you can about whooping cough and the technologies available today to protect your child from a preventable disease, whether it's whooping cough, measles, mumps, or any other common childhood disease.
Also keep in mind that the efficacy of immunization rarely provides lifelong immunity. Talk to your pediatrician about whooping cough, your child's risk of contracting it, as well as the benefits and drawbacks of the vaccines.

Remember, the more you know, the more you are able to make a knowledgeable, educated decision or decisions regarding your child's health, not only in relation to whooping cough, but other illnesses and disease processes.

We encourage parents or anyone providing care for children to take it upon themselves to further educate themselves regarding childhood diseases, the process involved in creating vaccinations, and most importantly, to study the safety and efficacy of vaccinations.

Do what you can to protect your children and keep them safe. Whether you decide to immunize or not, be aware of the signs and symptoms of whooping cough so that if your child comes down with symptoms, you can take steps earlier rather than later that will help reduce the severity and duration of the disease.